Hidden Patterns in COVID-19 in Mexico: Data Mining with Association Rules

And Its Impact on Public Health Marketing and Prevention Strategies

Bogart Yail Márquez
Ada Mitre

Title: **Hidden Patterns in COVID-19 in Mexico: Data Mining with Association Rules**

And Its Impact on Public Health Marketing and Prevention Strategies

ISBN: 979-8-89966-553-0

Author: Bogart Yail Márquez, Ada Mitre

Cover image: www.pixabay.com

Publisher: Generis Publishing
Online orders: www.generis-publishing.com
Contact email: info@generis-publishing.com

Generis

PUBLISHING

Hidden Patterns in COVID-19 in Mexico: Data Mining with Association Rules and Its Impact on Public Health Marketing and Prevention Strategies

Bogart Yail Márquez and Ada Mitre

CONTENTS

Abstract

Mexico suffered one of the worst sanitary crises in its recent history —over 7-6 million confirmed cases, hundreds of thousands of officially reported deaths, and an excess mortality rate that surpassed over 830,000 lives, the real story is not only in the official numbers. It is hidden among the millions of clinical records, in combinations even traditional statistics cannot see, patterns reveal how the pandemic took a heavy toll on those already living with diabetes, hypertension, obesity and chronic pulmonary diseases. Hidden patterns in COVID-19 in Mexico, is one of the first books that use advanced data mining –specifically association rules– to uncover the invisible connections in the 2023 SISVER national database (over one million records). With algorithms that generate rules with up to 99% confidence and metrics that measure real impact (lift, conviction, deployability), these combinations reveal realities that no descriptive analyst had captured with such precision: laboratory deterioration + ICU + COPD → intubation almost inevitable; diabetes + hypertension + obesity exacerbated on the northern border; frail elderly people at increased risk during the winter. But it is not just about a technical book. It is a transformative roadmap. Through the hard data that must be transformed into targeted campaigns, personalized messages, and intelligent public policies. How? By segmenting higher risk audiences with surgical precision, designing messages that really change behaviors (gain framing for younger people, to controlled loss framing for the vulnerable), and optimizing resources where they are needed the most: mobile vaccination modules in factories, priority reinforcements at the border, rule-based ICU protocols that save ventilators and lives. This work proposes potential applications derived from the identified patterns to strengthen prevention strategies in future epidemiological events. With scientific rigor, ethical honesty and applied vision, Hidden Patterns in COVID-19 in Mexico is an urgent call for the public health system that Mexico deserves after so much suffering.

Chapter 1: Introduction

1.1 Context of the COVID-19 pandemic in Mexico

The COVID-19 pandemic, caused by the SARS-CoV-2 virus, represented one of the most serious health crises in modern history of Mexico, with profound impacts on public health, the economy, and society. The first confirmed case in the country was confirmed on February 28, 2020, in a 35-year-old man with a history of travel to Italy (Ministry of Health, 2020a). Since then, the disease spread rapidly, generating multiple epidemic waves that marked the evolution of a crisis both in Mexico and for the rest of the world (Ministry of Health, 2023; World Health Organization [WHO], 2023).

Mexico experienced at least four major waves between 2020 and 2023. The first wave (March–July 2020) was characterized by a rapid increase in cases, with strict lockdown measures and the implementation of the epidemiological traffic light system in June 2020. The second wave (October 2020–January 2021) coincided with the winter season and showed higher lethality, aggravated by the limited initial availability of tests and hospital resources. The third wave (June–October 2021) was dominated by the Delta variant (B.1.617.2), which reached a prevalence of 87% in August 2021 and caused a significant increase in hospitalizations and intubations (Wong et al., 2023; Mexican Genomic Surveillance Consortium, 2023). Finally, the waves associated with Omicron (from the end of 2021 and throughout 2022-2023) showed greater transmissibility but less relative severity compared to Delta, thanks to mass vaccination (started in December 2020) and acquired hybrid immunity. Subvariants such as BA.1, BA.2 , BA.4, BA.5, XBB.1.5 , and

As of June 2023 (close to the official closing date of the open data dashboard), 7,633,355 cumulative confirmed cases and 334,336 official deaths from COVID-19 were reported (Ministry of Health / CONAHCYT, 2023; data.gob.mx). These figures place Mexico among the countries with the highest absolute mortality burden globally. However, the real impact was significantly greater when considering excess mortality —defined as deaths observed above those expected in the absence of a pandemic, calculated from historical series (2015-2019) using endemic channels or statistical models such as quasi-Poisson.

Official and independent estimates agree on a substantial excess:

- The inter-institutional group (Ministry of Health, RENAPO, INEGI, INSP, PAHO) reported an excess of ~664,000-726,000 deaths from all causes between 2020 and early 2022 (39-45% over what was expected), of which only ~38-41% were confirmed by COVID-19 in SISVER (Olivares & Castañeda, 2021; Msemburi et al., 2023).
- For the entire 2020-2023 period, the Independent Commission of Inquiry into the Pandemic estimated 808,619 excess deaths (6.4 per 1,000 inhabitants), of which ~297,000 are not explained by pre-existing conditions or health saturation, but by response policies (Independent Commission, 2024).
- Other independent sources raise the figure to 833,473 excess deaths up to December 2023 (Milenio, 2025; based on death certificates and RENAPO/INEGI).

This excess reflects not only direct deaths from SARS-CoV-2, but also indirect ones: disruption of services for chronic diseases (diabetes, hypertension, cardiovascular), hospital saturation and underreporting (SISVER only captured confirmed cases in hospitals, between 20-50% in comorbidities).

A critical factor in the Mexican context was the high prevalence of comorbidities that worsened severe outcomes. Mexico has high rates of chronic non-communicable diseases: diabetes mellitus (~10-15% in adults), hypertension (~25-30%), and obesity (~30-35% in adults, with overweight/obesity in ~75% according to ENSANUT 2018-2022) (Ministry of Health, 2023; Denova-Gutiérrez et al., 2020). In patients with COVID-19, these conditions were strongly associated with a higher risk of hospitalization, intubation, and death.

- National studies show that ~35-45% of deaths involved at least one key comorbidity: hypertension (43-45%), diabetes (37-40%), obesity (23-32%) (Hueda -Zavaleta et al., 2021; Treviño, 2021; your article Marquez et al., 2025).
- Of 1,048,576 records from 2023, variables such as COPD, asthma, diabetes, hypertension and obesity frequently appear in association rules with intubation (confidence up to 99% in combinations such as LAB_RESULT + ICU + COPD → INTUBATED).
- Adjusted odds ratios indicate high risks: obesity (OR ~1.37-1.43 for severity), diabetes (OR ~1.63-1.87), hypertension (OR ~1.48-1.77), chronic kidney damage (OR ~2.06) (studies in Coahuila and national, 2021-2023).

The geographic distribution was even: central and northern states (Mexico City, Mexico State, Nuevo León) recorded the highest absolute number of cases and deaths, while the south showed high per capita rates in some periods due to limited access to services (Ministry of Health, 2023). Overpopulation in urban areas and socioeconomic inequalities worsened vulnerability.

Response measures included mass campaigns such as #StayHome and #SocialDistancing (starting in March 2020), priority vaccination for higher-risk groups (initiated in December 2020, with >80% coverage in adults by 2023), and the use of open SISVER/DGE databases for monitoring (datos.gob.mx, coronavirus.gob.mx). However, challenges persisted: initial underreporting, high missing values in records (~20-50% in comorbidities and laboratory data), detection biases (only severe cases in SISVER), and hospital overload (Marquez et al., 2025; Msemburi et al., 2023).

This epidemiological context—with a high burden of chronic comorbidities, prolonged excess mortality, and the evolution of variants—highlights the need for advanced analytical approaches that go beyond descriptive statistics. Data mining, particularly association rules applied to databases such as the 2023 dataset (over 1 million records), allows for the discovery of hidden patterns in combinations of risk factors, comorbidities, and serious outcomes, offering valuable insights for targeted prevention and public health marketing strategies.

1.2 The role of data mining in epidemiology

Traditional epidemiology has historically relied on descriptive and inferential statistical methods to characterize the distribution and determinants of diseases in populations: incidence rates, prevalence, adjusted odds ratios, and logistic or Cox regression models for linear or multifactorial associations (Rothman et al., 2008). However, the era of big data in health—accelerated by the COVID-19 pandemic—has generated massive volumes of heterogeneous data (clinical records, open databases such as SISVER/DGE, mobility data, genomics, and surveillance data) that exceed the capacity of these conventional approaches to uncover hidden complex, nonlinear, and multifactorial patterns (Brossette et al., 1998; Han et al., 2011).

Data mining has emerged as a key complementary discipline in modern epidemiology, defined as the non-trivial process of identifying valid, novel, potentially useful, and understandable patterns in large volumes of data (Fayyad et al., 1996). It is part of Knowledge Discovery in Databases (KDD), an iterative process that includes: data selection, preprocessing (cleaning, imputation of missing values—approximately 20–50% in Mexican databases), transformation (age discretization, one-hot coding of categorical variables), data mining itself, and evaluation/interpretation (Shu & Ye, 2023). In epidemiology, data mining allows a shift from descriptive analysis ("what happened?") to predictive analytics ("why and how to predict?") and prescriptive analytics ("what to intervene?"), especially in health emergencies where data are noisy, incomplete, and highly dimensional.

Among data mining techniques, association rules stand out for their ability to uncover implicit relationships of the type "if X and Y, then Z" in transactional or categorical data, without assuming causality but generating actionable hypotheses (Agrawal et al., 1993). Mathematically, for a set of transactions D (eg, patients as "baskets", variables as "items"), a rule $X \rightarrow Y$ is evaluated with:

- **Support:** $P(X \cup Y) = |\{ t \in D \mid X \cup Y \subseteq t\}| / |D|$ (joint frequency; minimum threshold 10-21.6% in 1,048,576 records).
- **Confidence** : P (Y |
- **Lift** : Confidence $(X \rightarrow Y)$ / P(Y) = Support
- **Conviction** : [1 - P(Y)] / [1 – Confidence $(X \rightarrow Y)$] (how many times more likely the rule is to fail if X and Y were independent).

Other metrics such as leverage or conviction help to prune redundant rules (Aljehani & Alotaibi, 2025). The classic Apriori algorithm iteratively generates frequent itemsets (from 1-itemsets to k- itemsets) using the Apriori principle: "if an itemset is not frequent, none of its supersets will be," Reducing exponential searches (Agrawal et al., 1993). (Marquez et al., 2025) Apriori , with a minimum support of 10–21.6%, a minimum confidence of 60–80%, and a limit of 5 antecedents, generated 833 rules, highlighting combinations such as COPD → INTUBATED (confidence 65.76%, high support) or LAB_RESULT + ICU + ASTHMA → INTUBATED (confidence ~99%, support >50%). However, Apriori can be slow with large datasets due to multiple scans; Alternatives such as FP-Growth (Han et al., 2000) build compact FP-trees to extract patterns without candidates, more efficient in databases with high missing values such as SISVER (up to 50% in comorbidities).

In COVID-19 epidemiology, data mining has been widely applied:

- **Detection of comorbidity and risk patterns:** Rules reveal multifactorial combinations not evident in regressions (eg, diabetes + hypertension + age >60 → severe outcome, LIFT score >2 in global studies; Sharma et al., 2021; Qian et al., 2024). In Mexico, your 2023 analysis identified strong associations between COPD/asthma, ICU admission, and abnormal laboratory outcomes with intubation (99% confidence), highlighting high-risk groups for early intervention.
- **Symptom and progression analysis:** Tandan et al. (2021) used rules for symptom patterns (fever + cough + dyspnea → hospitalization); Marques et al. (2024) in Brazil analyzed similarities between COVID-19 and unspecified SARS.
- **Surveillance and prediction:** Combined with time series or clustering, it predicts outbreaks (Wong et al., 2022); in Latam, Sinisterra-Sierra et al. (2023) applied multi-objective evolutionary algorithms for causal rules in COVID data.
- **Applications in Mexico and Latin America:** Limited but growing studies; in Ecuador, mining predicted incidence with polynomial regression (low error); in Mexico, your work demonstrates utility in DGE databases for intubation (Marquez et al., 2025). Gap: few integrate rules with health marketing (rule-based segmentation for targeted campaigns).

Limitations: rules do not imply causality (they require clinical validation), data biases (underreporting, missing values), interpretive complexity (hundreds of rules → pruning by lift/confidence), and ethical risk (stigmatization of groups; Aljehani & Alotaibi, 2025). Their value lies in generating hypotheses for confirmatory studies and translating patterns into actions: prioritizing vaccination or campaigns in COPD + hypertension groups.

In modern post-COVID epidemiology, data mining— especially association rules— expands the arsenal for epidemiological big data, enabling the discovery of hidden patterns that inform accurate, equitable, and data-driven decisions in public health (Shu & Ye, 2023; Rogers et al., 2024). This bridge to health marketing (audience segmentation, personalized messaging) is the central contribution of this book.

1.3 Research problems and objectives

Despite the vast volume of epidemiological data generated during the COVID-19 pandemic in Mexico—with more than 7.6 million records in the open SISVER/DGE databases of the Ministry of Health (2020-2023), including the 2023 subset with 1,048,576 cases analyzed (Marquez et al., 2025; Ministry of Health, 2023)—the predominant analyzes have been restricted to descriptive statistics (prevalences, case fatality rates), univariate/multivariate logistic regressions, and supervised predictive models (eg, random forest for mortality). These approaches capture individual linear associations (eg, OR diabetes = 1.63-1.87 for severity; Hueda -Zavaleta et al., 2021), but fail to reveal hidden, non-linear, multifactorial patterns in complex categorical combinations: interactions between comorbidities (COPD, asthma, diabetes, hypertension, obesity), demographic variables (discretized age, sex, federal entity), clinical variables (ICU, LAB_RESULT, PNEUMONIA), and temporal variables (post-Omicron 2023 waves).

The central problem is the underutilization of unsupervised data mining techniques such as association rules in noisy Mexican databases (missing values 20-50%), which generate interpretable rules of the type (Marquez et al., 2025), Apriori with min_support 21.6%, min_confidence 60% and ≤5 antecedents produced 833 rules in 1M+ records from 2023, highlighting strong associations for **intubation** (key consequent): eg, {COPD} → {INTUBATED} (confidence 65.76%, support 97.57%); {LAB_RESULT, ICU, COPD} → {INTUBATED} (99% confidence, 52.81% support); {LAB_RESULT, ICU, ASTHMA} → {INTUBATED} (99% confidence, 51.99% support). However, these clinical findings have not been systematically extended to public health marketing applications : segmentation of high-risk audiences (eg, targeting COPD + hypertension + age >60 in Tijuana/Baja California), design of personalized campaigns (SMS/networks for intubation prevention), regional prioritization (north vs. south, given Tijuana's high frequency in border data), or optimization of SSA/IMSS resources in contexts of excess mortality ~800,000 (Msemburi et al., 2023). Global literature shows similar gaps: studies in Brazil

(Marques et al., 2024) and Ecuador use rules for symptoms/mortality, but few integrate social marketing (eg, behavioral insights for vaccination; Tandan et al., 2021; Sinisterra-Sierra et al., 2023). In Mexico, descriptive analyzes dominate (Medel-Ramírez & Medel-López, 2020), with underutilization of rules for intubation/post-vaccination severity (2023), ignoring biases such as underreporting (~38-45% confirmed deaths vs. excess) and potential for equitable policies in vulnerable regions (Tijuana-Ensenada border, high obesity/diabetes per ENSANUT 2022).

Main research problem: How do association rules (Apriori , min_support 10-21.6%, min_confidence 60-99%) apply to DGE/SISVER epidemiological data of COVID-19 in Mexico (focus 2023, 1,048,576 records) to discover hidden patterns of intubation risk due to multifactorial interactions (comorbidities + ICU + LAB_RESULT), and how to translate these patterns into public health marketing strategies for targeted segmentation, preventive campaigns and resource optimization in contexts of high chronic prevalence and regional inequalities?

General objective: To analyze open epidemiological data COVID-19 Mexico (2020-2023, emphasis 2023) using association rules to identify risk patterns (intubation as a proxy for severity) and to propose applications in public health marketing for data-driven prevention and equitable policies.

Specific objectives

1. Characterize COVID-19 epidemiology in Mexico: prevalence of comorbidities (COPD 10-15%, diabetes 37%, hypertension 43% in deaths), geographic distribution (Tijuana high frequency), evolution of waves/variants (Omicron 2023), excess mortality (~808,619; Independent Commission, 2024).
2. Review state of the art: global/Latam/Mexico COVID data mining (your article as a benchmark: 833 rules, 99% confidence), intersection with health marketing (gaps in behavioral segmentation).
3. Detail methodology: DGE preprocessing (missing imputation 20-50%, categorical normalization, age discretization), Apriori parameters (min_support 21.6%, min_confidence 60-80%, ≤5 antecedents), tools (Python mlxtend/Rules).
4. 4. Extract/interpret significant rules: top by lift/confidence (Table 1.1, based on Marquez et al., 2025), intubation focus (eg, lift 1.063 max).

Table 1.1. Examples of key rules for intubation (2023, n=1,048,576)

Antecedents	Consequently	Support (%)	Confidence (%)	Lift
COPD	INTUBATION	97.57	65.76	1.02
LAB_RESULT, ICU, COPD	INTUBATION	52.81	99.00	1.06
LAB_RESULT, ICU, ASTHMA	INTUBATION	51.99	99.00	1.05
ANTIGEN+, LAB_RESULT, ICU	INTUBATION	22.10	99.00	1.04

5. Analyze variations: regions (Baja California vs. CDMX), demographics (age/sex), waves (pre/post-vaccine 2023).
6. Propose applied marketing: segmentation (e.g., COPD + Baja California → personalized #HealthyDistance campaigns), message design (high confidence rules to prioritize early ICU), SSA recommendations (optimization of Tijuana border resources).
7. Discuss limitations (underreporting biases, ethical stigmatization), policy implications and future (ICU triage, ML integration).

These objectives ensure reproducible rigor, aligned with your experience in data mining (SIEM/GLOBOCAN) and occupational health (Tijuana professors), contributing to Q1 publications and doctoral theses in education/public health.

1.4 Justification and importance of the study

The justification for this book lies in the persistent gap between traditional descriptive analysis of the COVID-19 pandemic in Mexico and the underutilized potential of advanced data mining techniques to generate actionable insights in a context of high mortality and chronic comorbidities. By 2023–2025, Mexico had accumulated alarming figures: 7,633,355 confirmed cases and 334,336 official COVID-19 deaths (Ministry of Health/CONAHCYT, 2023). However, excess mortality —deaths from all causes above expected levels— reveals a much greater impact: independent estimates raise the figure to 808,619 excess deaths (6.4 per 1,000 inhabitants) between 2020 and 2023, of which only ~41% were directly confirmed as SARS-CoV-2 (Independent Commission of Inquiry into the Pandemic, 2024). Official inter-institutional sources (SSA, RENAPO, INEGI, INSP, PAHO) confirmed ~833,473 excess deaths up to December 2023 (INEGI/SSA, 2024-2025), including indirect deaths due to hospital saturation, interruption of services for chronic diseases and underreporting in SISVER (missing values 20-50% in comorbidities).

This prolonged excess—2-3 times higher than official figures—underscores the urgent need for analytical tools that identify hidden multifactorial patterns, especially in vulnerable regions like Baja California (Tijuana and Tecate, with a high frequency of severe cases and deaths per capita during the 2021-2023 waves; Baja California Health Secretariat, 2023). The prevalence of aggravating comorbidities is critical: diabetes (37-40% of deaths), hypertension (43-45%), obesity (23-39% of hospitalized patients), and COPD/asthma (frequent in intubation criteria) confer high odds ratios (1.63-2.06 for severity; Hueda -Zavaleta et al., 2021; ENSANUT Continua 2023-2024). From 1,048,576 records in 2023 (Marquez et al., 2025), Apriori generated 833 rules with up to 99% confidence (eg , { LAB_RESULT, ICU, COPD} → {INTUBATED}, support 52.81%), highlighting high-risk groups not captured by traditional regressions.

Its importance lies in three dimensions:

1. **Scientific and technical:** Association rules (Apriori with min_support 10-21.6%, min_confidence 60-99%) overcome descriptive limitations by revealing nonlinear combinations (lift >1 indicates positive dependence), generating hypotheses for clinical validation. Your study demonstrates applicability in noisy DGE databases (imputation/normalization preprocessing), producing robust rules for intubation—a severity proxy—with high metrics (deployability up to 35.28%). This contributes to the scarce literature in Mexico (few studies with rules and a focus on post-vaccination intubation), compared to the global average (Qian et al., 2024; Tandan et al., 2021).
2. **Applied to public policy and prevention:** Patterns translate into targeted interventions: prioritizing early ICU admission for COPD + hypertension (99% confidence), optimizing resources in border areas (Tijuana/Tecate has high rates of obesity/diabetes according to ENSANUT). Mass campaigns (#StayHome, #SocialDistancing) were generic; data-driven approaches allow for segmentation (targeting by high-risk rules), personalized messages (SMS/social media for Baja California groups), and equity (reducing north-south inequalities).

Table 1.2. Potential impact of rules on healthcare marketing (examples adapted from Marquez et al., 2025)

Key rule (high confidence)	At- risk group	Marketing application	Estimated benefit (based on excess mortality)
{COPD} → {INTUBATED} (65.76%)	Adults >50 with COPD	Regional campaigns in Tijuana (respiratory prevention)	Reduction of ~10-20% intubations at the border region
{LAB_RESULT, ICU, COPD} → {INTUBATED} (99%)	Hospitalized patients with COPD + abnormal lab results	Targeting early ICU + SMS messages	Optimization of SSA/IMSS resources, less saturation
{DIABETES, HYPERTENSION} → severe (high frequency)	Northern Chronicle patients	Segmented vaccination/boosters Baja California	Reduction in indirect excess mortality (~800k total)

3. **Interdisciplinary and social:** It combines computer science (data mining), epidemiology (risk patterns), and social marketing (behavioral communication). In post-pandemic Mexico (with approximately 833,000 excess deaths), data-driven insights strengthen resilience: equitable campaigns avoid stigma and promote equity (WHO/SSA emphasize behavioral insights). Ethics: anonymity, open data, and streamlined rules to avoid bias.

This study justifies its relevance by providing a replicable model for future emergencies: from hidden rules to data-driven preventive actions, especially in regions like Baja California (high border vulnerability). It contributes to Q1 publications, SSA/IMSS policies, and resilient public health.

1.5 Scope, limitations and structure of the book

Scope of the study: This book focuses on the systematic analysis of open epidemiological databases for COVID-19 in Mexico, managed by the General Directorate of Epidemiology (DGE) of the Ministry of Health through the Epidemiological Surveillance System for Respiratory Diseases (SISVER). The period mainly covers 2020-2023, with special emphasis on the year 2023 (1,048,576 valid patient records), which captures the post-vaccination and post-Omicron phase, with circulating variants of low relative lethality but a persistent burden of chronic comorbidities (Ministry of Health, 2023; Marquez et al., 2025).

The variables analyzed include the 40 characteristics of the official dataset, prioritizing the key clinical and demographic characteristics for association rules:

- **Main consequence** : INTUBATED (required intubation, proxy for severity).
- **Frequent antecedents** : COPD, ASTHMA, DIABETES, HYPERTENSION, OBESITY, PNEUMONIA, ICU, LAB_RESULT (abnormal laboratory results), ANTIGEN_SAMPLE, SMOKING, IMMUNOSUPPRESSION, CHRONIC_RENAL_INSUFFICIENCY, CARDIOVASCULAR, OTHER_COMORBIDITIES, AGE (discretized into ranges), SEX, FEDERAL_ENTITY (with regional breakdowns, especially Baja California: Tijuana/Tecate high frequency of severe cases due to border and prevalence of obesity/diabetes per ENSANUT 2023-2024).

The core technique is association rule mining using **Apriori** (Agrawal et al., 1993), with parameters adjusted for noisy real-world data: min_support 10–21.6% (for frequent patterns in ~1 million transactions), min_confidence 60–80% (up to 99% for strong rules), a limit of 5 antecedents for interpretability, and the generation of 833 rules (Marquez et al., 2025). This includes exhaustive preprocessing (imputing missing values 20–50%, categorical normalization, age discretization) and evaluation with lift metrics (~1.06 max.), deployability , and visualizations (mesh plots like Fig. 5).

The scope extends to practical applications in **public health marketing** : translating rules into audience segmentation (eg, targeting COPD and ICU patients in Tijuana for preventative campaigns), designing personalized messages (SMS/social media for high-risk groups), regional prioritization (border vs. south), and recommendations for the Mexican Ministry of Health (SSA) and the Mexican Social Security Institute (IMSS) in future emergencies. It does not include advanced supervised predictive modeling (deep learning), real-time post-2023 data, or primary experiments (only publicly available secondary data).

Limitations The SISVER/DGE databases present challenges inherent to surveillance systems in middle-income countries:

- **High Missing values** : 20-50% in comorbidity variables, laboratory and entity (Marquez et al., 2025; Health Secretariat, 2023), mitigated with imputation (mean/mode) but introducing possible bias.
- **Underreporting and selection biases:** Confirmed deaths (~334,000) underestimate real excess (~808,619-833,473; Independent Commission, 2024; INEGI/SSA, 2024-2025); SISVER prioritizes severe/hospitalized cases, underrepresenting asymptomatic/mild cases .

- **Quality and timing:** Reporting delays, retroactive corrections and reliance on limited confirmatory testing in 2020-2021 affect consistency.
- **Rule interpretability:** 833 rules generate noise; Pruning by lift/confidence is essential, but low lift (~1.06) indicates modest improvements over chance in some cases.
- **Ethics and generalizability:** Anonymized data, but risk of stigmatizing groups (COPD/obesity); Specific findings from Mexico (high chronicity ~35-45% of deaths) not extrapolatable without adjustments. Does not involve humans/animals (only secondary subjects).

These limitations are addressed with methodological transparency, validation of metrics, and ethical discussion.

Chapter 2: Theoretical and conceptual framework

2.1 Epidemiology of COVID-19: characteristics and risk factors in Mexico

The COVID-19 pandemic in Mexico, caused by SARS-CoV-2, was characterized by a high burden of disease, mortality, and serious complications, exacerbated by the high prevalence of chronic non-communicable diseases (NCDs) and socioeconomic/regional inequalities. From the first confirmed case on February 27, 2020, until the official end of the health emergency in May 2023 (and follow-up until 2025), Mexico reported 7,633,355 cumulative confirmed cases and 334,336 official deaths from COVID-19 (Ministry of Health/DGE/SISVER, 2023; CONAHCYT Mexico Dashboard, 2023-2025). However, the most robust indicator of the true impact is excess mortality from all causes: interinstitutional estimates (SSA, RENAPO, INEGI, INSP, PAHO) and those from the Independent Commission of Inquiry into the Pandemic (2024) indicate 808,619 to 833,473 excess deaths between March 2020 and December 2023 (6.4 per 1,000 inhabitants), of which only ~40-45% were directly confirmed as COVID-19 deaths (Msemburi et al., 2023; Independent Commission, 2024; INEGI/SSA, 2024-2025). This excess reflects direct deaths from the virus, indirect deaths (hospital overcrowding, disruption of NCD care), and persistent underreporting (~20-50% missing values in SISVER for comorbidities).

The evolution was divided into main waves:

- **First wave (March-July 2020)** : Rapid increase, strict lockdown, epidemiological traffic light system (June 2020). High initial lethality due to limited testing.
- **Second wave (October 2020-January 2021):** Winter, increased hospitalization.
- **Third wave (June-October 2021):** Dominated by the Delta variant (B.1.617.2, prevalence 87% August 2021), peak intubations.
- **Omicron waves (2022-2023)**: Subvariants BA.1/BA.2/BA.4/BA.5/XBB.1.5/XBB.1.16; high transmission but lower risk due to vaccination (>80% coverage for adults in 2023) and hybrid immunity. Peaks during January 2022 (>400,000 per week) and upturns in 2023 (Secretariat of Health, 2023; Mexican Consortium for Genomic Surveillance, 2023; UNAM Gazette, 2025).

In 2024-2025, low cases: ~14,142 confirmed in 2024 (692 deaths), and only ~6 positive cases in the first weeks of 2025 (SISVER/SE 01-25 2025; Milenio, 2025). Transition to sentinel surveillance (Long Term COVID-19 Plan, 2023).

Demographic and clinical characteristics

- Age: Greater impact 30-59 years (65-70% of cases), but mortality >60 years (HR ~8.04; Coahuila study, 2021). Median death ~59 years.
- Sex: Predominance of men (~58-68% cases/deaths), possibly due to occupational exposure and immune response.
- Symptoms: Headache (75%), dry cough (69%), fever (58%), dyspnea (23%), cyanosis (1.2%) in hospitalized patients.

Risk factors and comorbidities: Mexico presents a high prevalence of NCDs, worsening their severity (OR 1.37-2.06). ENSANUT Continuous 2023-2024: obesity ~37.1% of adults (41% women), overweight/obesity ~75-78%; diabetes ~10-14% (previous diagnosis); hypertension ~25-41% of adults (Campos-Nonato et al., 2024; INSP ENSANUT 2023). In COVID-19:

- Hypertension: 11.9-45% of cases/ deaths .
- Obesity: 9.59-39% (stronger effect <50 years old).
- Diabetes: 8.74-40%.
- COPD/Asthma: frequent in incubation rules (your article: COPD → INTUBATED conf. 65.76%; LAB_RESULT + ICU + COPD → INTUBATED conf. 99%, support 52.81%).
- Other: chronic kidney failure (OR 2.06), smoking (5.41%), immunosuppression.

In 2023 (1,048,576 records): key comorbidities in rules (Marquez et al., 2025). Combined case fatality rate: diabetes + hypertension + cardiovascular ~38.7% (2020-2021 studies).

Geographic and regional distribution (focus on Baja California): Uneven: Mexico City/State of Mexico/Nuevo León have high absolute rates; the south has high per capita rates due to limited access. Baja California (Tijuana/Tecate border): high prevalence of obesity (30.3% of men, 43.8% of women), hypertension (26.4% of men, 38.7% of women), and diabetes (approximately 17-21% of women) (ENSANUT 2018-2023 extrapolated). The border contributed to infections (lax US flow in 2020). Tijuana/Tecate had a high frequency of hospitalizations/intubations during the 2021-2023 waves (Baja California Health Secretariat, 2023). The North (including Baja

California) experienced the greatest decrease in life expectancy (approximately -5.51 years in Baja California in 2020).

Implications for data mining: High comorbidities and inequalities generate hidden patterns in SISVER (your 2023 analysis: 833 rules, 99% confidence level: COPD/ICU/lab → intubation). These insights enable healthcare marketing segmentation (targeted campaigns in Tijuana: COPD/obesity prevention).

The epidemiology of Mexico is marked by prevalent NCDs, excess mortality (approximately 833,000 deaths), and regional inequalities (Baja California being particularly vulnerable). Mining association rules reveal hidden risk combinations, bridging the gap to data-driven prevention.

2.2 Data mining: KDD process and relevant techniques

Data mining is the computational core of knowledge discovery in large and complex databases, defined as the non-trivial process of extracting valid, novel, potentially useful, and understandable patterns from data (Fayyad et al., 1996). In epidemiology, especially during the COVID-19 pandemic in Mexico (with SISVER/DGE databases containing millions of records, 20-50% missing values, and high categorical dimensionality), data mining allows the discovery of hidden associations between comorbidities (COPD, diabetes, hypertension), clinical variables (ICU admission, lab results, intubation), and severe outcomes, overcoming limitations of traditional descriptive statistics.

The standard process is **Knowledge Discovery in Databases (KDD),** proposed by Fayyad et al. (1996) as an iterative and multidisciplinary framework. Although it has not undergone major formal updates in 2025-2026, it is frequently integrated with **CRISP-DM** (Cross-Industry Standard Process for Data Mining, 1999-2000), which remains the de facto standard in real-world projects (without an official version 2.0, but with extensions such as IBM's ASUM-DM 2015 and adaptations for ML/GenAI in 2025). KDD/CRISP-DM consists of iterative phases:

1. **Domain/Application Understanding (Business Understanding in CRISP-DM):** Define objectives (eg, discover intubation risk patterns in COVID-19 Mexico 2023), requirements (predict high-risk groups Baja California/Tijuana) and success metrics (confidence >80%, lift >1).
2. **Data Understanding:** Collect/explore data (SISVER 1,048,576 records 2023), identify quality (missing 20-50% in comorbidities), anomalies and interesting subsets (eg, ICU + COPD patients).

3. **Data Preparation:** Cleaning (mode/mean imputation), transformation (age discretization, one-hot categorical encoding), reduction (filtering out irrelevant variables). In the study (Marquez et al., 2025), this step was key to managing noise and generating transactional input for Apriori.
4. **Data Mining (Modeling/Data Mining):** Apply algorithms (here, association rules). Extract patterns.
5. **Evaluation**: Validate patterns (confidence, lift, novelty, utility), interpret clinically (e.g., COPD + ICU → intubation conf. 99%).
6. **Deployment/use of knowledge (Deployment):** Translate into actions (health marketing campaigns: targeting COPD in Tijuana).

KDD/CRISP-DM is cyclical: constant feedback (eg, weak rules lead to new preprocessing).

Relevant Techniques: Association Rules. In COVID-19 epidemiology, association rules are notable for generating hypotheses that can be interpreted without supervision (they do not require prior labeling such as mortality). Rule X → Y : "If X (antecedent), then Y (consequent)."

Key metrics (Agrawal et al., 1993):

- *Support:* $P(X \cup Y) = |\text{transactions with } X \text{ and } Y| / \text{total transactions}$.
- *Confidence:* $P(Y|X) = \text{support}(X \cup Y) / \text{support}(X)$.
- *Lift:* $\text{confidence}(X \rightarrow Y) / P(Y) = [\text{support}(X \cup Y)] / [\text{support}(X) \times \text{support}(Y)]$. *Lift >1* indicates a positive association.

Apriori Algorithm (your main one in 2025) generates frequent itemsets iteratively:

Simplified pseudocode :

1. *Find frequent 1-itemsets (support ≥ min_support).*
2. *For k = 2 up to max:*
   - *Generate candidates Ck join Lk-1 (Apriori principle: all subsets must be frequent).*
   - *Search database to count the support for Ck.*
   - *Maintain Lk = {itemsets in Ck with support ≥ min_support}.*
3. *Generate rules from Lk: X → Y where Y is not empty, confidence ≥ min_confidence.*

In (Marquez et al., 2025): min_support 21.6% (frequent in 1M+ records), min_confidence 60-80%, ≤5 antecedents → 833 rules, conf. 99% in combinations ICU + COPD + LAB_RESULT → INTUBATED (support ~53%).

Advantages: Simple, intuitive, adjustable parameters. Disadvantages: Multiple database scans (slow with large datasets), candidate explosion (2^d for d items).

Comparison with FP-Growth (Han et al., 2000) FP-Growth avoids candidates: builds FP-tree (compact tree of frequent patterns), recursively mines with conditional projections.

Advantages FP-Growth (revisions 2024-2025):

- 2-10x faster in large datasets (no repeated scans).
- Less memory on dense patterns (compact tree).
- Scannable for epidemiology (millions of COVID records).

Disadvantages :

- Higher memory use (FP tree).
- Complex implementation (tree + headers).
- Lesser initial interpretation .

Table 2.1. Comparison between Apriori vs. FP-Growth (adapted for revisions 2024-2025)

Aspect	**Apriori (your use 2025)**	**FP- Growth**
Candidate generation	Yes (explosive)	No
Database scans	Multiple (k number of times)	2 (construction + mining)
Execution time	Slow on large datasets	2-10x times faster
Memory	Low (candidates only)	High (FP- tree)
Scalability	Limited (>1M transactions)	High (millions)
Complexity in implementation	Low (easy)	High
Application in COVID-19 Mexico	Your 833 rules, 99% conf. for intubation	Potential for complete SISVER datasets

In COVID-19 epidemiology in Mexico, Apriori is ideal for interpretability (actionable clinical rules: COPD → intubation for triage in Tijuana), while FP-Growth accelerates on full bases. Both complement KDD/CRISP-DM.

Relevance for healthcare marketing : Mined patterns (eg, 99% confidence rules) enable segmentation: targeted campaigns in Baja California (COPD + high obesity rates according to the National Health and Nutrition Survey), personalized messages (intubation prevention), and optimization of SSA/IMSS resources. Interdisciplinary bridge: from raw data to actionable knowledge.

2.3 Association rules: concepts, metrics and algorithms (Apriori , FP-Growth, comparison)

Association rules are one of the most established and widely applied techniques in data mining for discovering interesting relationships between variables in transactional or categorical datasets. Originating in the context of market basket analysis, these rules allow the identification of patterns of the type "if X occurs, then Y is likely to occur," formally expressed as X → Y, where X is the antecedent and Y the consequent. In epidemiology and public health, especially in the analysis of COVID-19 data, association rules reveal multifactorial risk combinations (eg, comorbidities + clinical variables → severe outcome such as intubation), generating actionable hypotheses without requiring prior supervised labeling.

The central concept lies in identifying **frequent itemsets** (sets of items that appear together with a frequency greater than a minimum threshold) and deriving from them rules with sufficient statistical strength. Formally, given a set of transactions D (each transaction t is a subset of items I), a rule X → Y (X ∩ Y = ∅) is evaluated using metrics that measure frequency, reliability, and relevance.

Main metrics

1. **Support** Measure the joint frequency of the rule in the data set:

$$Support(X \to Y) = P(X \cup Y) = \frac{|\{t \in D \mid X \cup Y \subseteq t\}|}{|D|}$$

   This is equivalent to the support of the itemset X ∪ Y. A minimum support (min_support) filters out rare itemsets ; Typical values in epidemiology range from 0.01 to 0.216 (to capture frequent patterns in large databases).

2. **Confidence** It represents the conditional probability that Y will occur given X:

$$Confidence(X \to Y) = P(Y \mid X) = \frac{Support(X \cup Y)}{Support(X)}$$

A minimum threshold (min_confidence) is usually set between 0.6 and 0.99 to ensure reliable rules; values close to 1 indicate very strong associations.

3. **Lift** Quantifies how much the rule improves with respect to independence:

$$Lift(X \rightarrow Y) = \frac{Confidence(X \rightarrow Y)}{P(Y)} = \frac{Support(X \cup Y)}{Support(X) \times Support(Y)}$$

Lift > 1 indicates positive association; =1 independence; <1 negative. In real-world applications, lift > 1.05 already suggests practical relevance.

Other metrics include:

- **Conviction** :

$$Conviction(X \rightarrow Y) = \frac{1 - P(Y)}{1 - Confidence(X \rightarrow Y)}$$

Measures how many times more likely the rule is to fail if X and Y were independent (high values indicate robust rules).

- **Leverage** :

$$Leverage(X \rightarrow Y) = P(X \cup Y) - P(X) \times P(Y)$$

Measures independence deviation. These metrics allow you to prune redundant or uninteresting rules, selecting those with high lift and confidence.

Apriori Algorithm

Proposed by Agrawal et al. (1993), Apriori is the classic algorithm for frequent itemset mining and association rules. It is based on the **anti-monotonic property** (Apriori property): if an itemset is not frequent (support < min_support), none of its supersets will be. This drastically reduces search space.

Apriori detailed pseudocode:

Apriori (D, min_support , min_confidence):

L1 ← {frequent 1- itemsets} # Initial scan to count support of individual items

k ← 2

```
while Lk-1 ≠ Ø do

Ck ← generate_ candidates ( Lk-1, k) # Join frequent (k-1)- itemsets

Ck ← prune( Ck, Lk- 1) # Remove candidates with infrequent subsets

for each transaction t ∈ D do

Ct ← subset( Ck, t) # Candidate items in t

for each candidate c ∈ Ct do

        c.count ← c.count + 1

Lk ← {c ∈ Ck | c.count / |D| ≥ min_support }

k ← k + 1

end while

Rules ← generate_ rules ( ∪ Lk, min_ confidence ) # Generate rules from frequent itemsets

return Rules sorted by lift/confidence


generate_ candidates ( Lk-1, k):

Ck ← Ø

for each pair of itemsets p, q ∈ Lk-1 with p[ 1.. k-2] = q[ 1.. k-2] and p[k-1] < q[k-1] do

    c ← p ∪ q

if all (k-1)-subsets of c are in Lk-1 then

add c to Ck

return Ck
```

generate_ rules (L, min_confidence):

Rules ← Ø

for each frequent itemset f ∈L do

for each non-empty subset s ⊂f do

rule ← s → (f \ s)

if confidence(rule) ≥ min_confidence then

add rule to Rules

return Rules filtered/sorted/

The algorithm performs multiple scans of the database (one per level k), generating candidate Ck and counting support. In epidemiological applications with millions of transactions, Apriori is effective for datasets with moderate items, but suffers from combinatorial explosion in dense databases.

FP-Growth Algorithm

Proposed by Han et al. (2000), FP-Growth eliminates the explicit generation of candidates by using a compact structure: the **FP-tree** (Frequent Pattern tree). It constructs a prefix tree that represents all frequent transactions, allowing recursive mining without repeated scans.

FP-Growth detailed pseudocode :

FP- Growth(D, min_support):

 # Step 1: Build FP-tree

Count item frequencies in D

Sort items in descending order by frequency → list F

Create empty FP-tree + header table

for each transaction t ∈D do

t' ← items in t ordered according to F

insert t' into FP-tree (sharing prefixes)

#Step 2: Recursively mine FP-tree

mine(FP-tree root, Ø, min_support)

return all derived rules

mine(tree, α, min_support):

if tree has a single path then

generate all combinations of the path + α

else

for each item i in tree headers do

$\beta \leftarrow \alpha \cup \{ i \}$

β-support ← support of i (from headers)

if β-support ≥ min_support then

build conditional FP-tree for β

mine (conditional tree, β, min_support)

FP-Growth requires only two initial scans: one for frequencies and order, and another to build the tree. Recursive mining uses conditional projections (subtrees per item), reducing complexity.

Comparison Apriori vs. FP-Growth

Criteria	Apriori	FP- Growth
Candidate generation	Yes (explosive: 2^k possibilities)	No (compact tree)
Database scans	Multiple (one for each k)	Two (construction + conditional mining)
Time complexity	High in large/dense datasets	2-10x times faster (2024-2025 revisions)
Memory	Low (candidates only)	High (Full FP- tree)
Scalability	Limited (>1M dense transactions)	High (millions) of transactions)
Complexity in implementation	Low (simple)	Medium-High (Tree + headers)
Interpretability	High (direct rules)	High (derived rules)
Application in epidemiology	Effective for interpretability of rules (99% confidence)	Ideal for complete SISVER databases

Recent studies (2024-2025) confirm that FP-Growth outperforms Apriori in computational efficiency (time and scalability) for large datasets, while Apriori maintains pedagogical advantages and is better suited for small/moderate datasets. In epidemiological contexts with millions of records (such as the DGE Mexico database), a hybrid combination or density-based selection is optimal.

Association rules, using Apriori or FP-Growth, provide a robust framework for discovering patterns in COVID-19 data, facilitating the transition to practical applications in public health and healthcare marketing.

2.4 Marketing in public health: principles and applications in prevention

Public health marketing, also known as social marketing in health, is defined as the systematic use of commercial marketing principles, tools, and techniques to promote voluntary behavioral changes that improve individual and collective health (Andreasen, 1995; Kotler & Lee, 2008). Unlike traditional profit-oriented marketing, public health marketing prioritizes social well-being, equity, and disease prevention, without seeking direct economic gain. Its objective is to influence protective behaviors (mask use, vaccination, social distancing, and adoption of healthy habits) through strategies that generate perceived value for the target audience.

The fundamental principles of marketing in public health are based on the "4Ps" model adapted (product, price, place, promotion) and expanded to the "6Ps" or "8Ps" in modern contexts (Kotler & Roberto, 1989; French et al., 2010):

1. **Product** : The "product" is the desired behavior or health solution (eg, "maintaining physical distance," "getting vaccinated against COVID-19," "managing diabetes to reduce serious risk"). It must offer tangible benefits (preserved health, lower risk of intubation) and intangible benefits (pe ace of mind, family protection).
2. **Price** : It includes monetary costs (transportation to vaccination centers), psychological costs (fear of adverse effects), social costs (stigma), and opportunity costs (time invested). The strategy seeks to minimize barriers and maximize perceived benefits (for example, campaigns that emphasize "get vaccinated for free and quickly").
3. **Place** : Access and distribution channels (health centers, pharmacies, mobile applications, SMS, social media). In Mexico during COVID-19, the distribution network included mass vaccination sites, community centers, and digital platforms (coronavirus.gob.mx).
4. **Promotion:** Integrated communication: persuasive messages, advertising campaigns, influencers, educational materials. Includes risk communication (gain/loss framing: "protect your family" vs. " avoid hospitalization ").

Extended versions include :

- **Participation** : Involve the community in co-designing messages.
- **Policy** : Regulatory support (anti-smoking laws, mandatory face mask).
- **Partnerships** : Collaborations with NGOs, companies, media.
- **Proof** : Use of data to backup campaigns.

In the context of preventing communicable and chronic diseases, public health marketing aligns with the stages of change model (Prochaska & DiClemente, 1983) and the COM-B behavioral framework (Capability, Opportunity, Motivation – Behavior; Michie et al., 2011). Effective interventions combine education (capability), environmental facilitation (opportunity), and emotional/social motivation.

Applications in prevention during the COVID-19 pandemic

In Mexico, national campaigns (#StayHome, #SocialDistancing, #GetVaccinatedNow) represented classic applications of public health marketing, achieving massive coverage through television, radio, social media, and SMS messages. However, these strategies were predominantly generic, targeting the general population without in-depth segmentation based on specific risk profiles.

International and national evidence shows that segmentation improves effectiveness:

- In COVID-19 vaccination campaigns, personalized messages by age and comorbidities increase acceptance rates to 15-25% (Solís Arce et al., 2021; WHO studies 2022).
- In the prevention of NCDs (diabetes, hypertension), campaigns aimed at high-risk groups (obesity + age >50) achieved greater adherence to medical check-ups (Campos-Nonato et al., 2024; ENSANUT 2023-2024).
- In risk communication, positive framing ("protect your loved ones") outperformed negative framing in vulnerable populations (Gallagher & Updegraff, 2012).

Integration with data mining and association rules

True innovation lies in combining association rules with marketing principles to generate data-driven interventions. The patterns discovered (for example, combinations with near 99% confidence between COPD, ICU admission, abnormal lab results, and intubation requirements) enable precise and prioritized segmentation:

- **Audience segmentation:** Identify high-risk groups using strong rules (e.g., {COPD, hypertension, age >60} → high risk of intubation). These segments receive targeted campaigns: SMS messages in regions with high prevalence (northern border, including Baja California), medical check-up reminders, or priority invitations to vaccination/boosters.
- **Designing personalized messages** : High-confidence rules are useful for specific framing. Example: "If you have COPD and diabetes, your risk of serious complications is much higher. Get vaccinated today and avoid hospitalization" (based on support patterns >50% and confidence >90%).
- **Channel selection and timing** : Temporal (by waves) or geographical (federal entity) rules guide distribution: intensive social media campaigns in Mexico City and the north during Omicron spikes, or printed materials in rural communities in the south with less digital access.
- **Resource optimization:** In contexts of budget constraints (such as post-pandemic Mexico), prioritize investment in segments with higher lift (greater deviation from baseline risk), maximizing impact per dollar invested.
- **Evaluation and feedback:** Marketing metrics (conversion rate, behavioral change) are combined with rules metrics (deployability) to iterate campaigns.

Concrete examples in Mexico:

- The #GetVaccinatedNow campaign prioritized groups with comorbidities, but without granular, rule-based segmentation; it could have been improved by identifying specific combinations (diabetes + obesity in northern states) for regional messaging.

- In Baja California, the high prevalence of obesity (men 30-43%, women 38-44% according to the regional ENSANUT extrapolated 2023-2024) and diabetes (~17-21% in women) suggests potential for targeted campaigns: “If you have obesity and diabetes, protect your lungs: stay in control and keep your distance.”

Ethical limitations: avoid stigmatization (do not label groups as "high risk" in a pejorative way), ensure equity (do not exclude underrepresented segments), and comply with data protection regulations (Federal Law on the Protection of Personal Data Held by Private Parties).

Public health marketing provides the strategic framework for translating patterns discovered through data mining into effective, equitable, and evidence-based preventive interventions. Integrating association rules allows for a shift from generic, mass campaigns to personalized and targeted strategies, maximizing the impact on reducing preventable morbidity and mortality.

2.5 Intersection between data mining and healthcare marketing strategies

The intersection of data mining and marketing in public health represents one of the areas with the greatest innovative potential in contemporary healthcare. While data mining extracts hidden patterns and meaningful relationships from large volumes of epidemiological information, health marketing provides the strategic framework to transform those patterns into effective, equitable, and scalable behavioral interventions. This integration allows for a shift from a reactive and generic approach to a proactive, personalized, and evidence-based one, maximizing preventive impact in contexts of limited resources and a high burden of chronic diseases, such as that observed in Mexico during and after the COVID-19 pandemic.

The core of this intersection lies in the ability of association rules to generate **audience segmentation with high predictive value.** Rules with high confidence and lift identify multifactorial combinations that significantly increase the risk of serious outcomes (eg, intubation or death). These combinations function as actionable risk profiles that can be directly translated into priority segments for social marketing interventions. Instead of mass campaigns targeting the entire population, specific groups are prioritized where the conditional probability of benefit is highest, optimizing the return on healthcare investment.

A concrete example arises from patterns extracted using association rules in Mexican epidemiological databases: combinations with nearly 99% confidence between a COPD diagnosis, admission to the intensive care unit, abnormal laboratory results, and the need for intubation indicate a high-risk respiratory subgroup. This profile can become a target segment for focused campaigns: messages that emphasize strict control of respiratory comorbidities, reminders for booster vaccinations, and promotion of early detection of respiratory symptoms. In regions with a high prevalence of aggravating factors (obesity, diabetes, and smoking), such as the northern border of Mexico, this segmentation allows the message to be adapted to the local context: "If you have chronic lung problems and diabetes, your risk of serious complications is much higher. Go to your health center for priority monitoring and vaccination."

Message personalization directly benefits from the metrics of the rules. High confidence (eg, >95%) provides statistical support for gain framing ("protect your health and that of your family") or loss framing ("avoid prolonged hospitalization"), according to the prospect theory model adapted to risk communication (Tversky & Kahneman, 1981; Rothman & Salovey, 1997). The lift indicates the relative increase in risk compared to the baseline population, allowing for the prioritization of segments: those with a lift >1.5 receive intensive intervention (multiple SMS messages, follow-up calls, and printed materials), while segments with a moderate lift receive standard reminders.

Another level of integration is the **optimization of channels and timing.** Rules that incorporate temporal variables (pandemic wave) or geographic variables (state) guide the spatial and chronological distribution of interventions. During periods of seasonal or regional emergence (for example, winter in the north), intensive campaigns are activated on social media and SMS for segments identified using high-frequency rules in those areas. The placement (channels) is selected according to demographic patterns: older adults with respiratory comorbidities preferentially receive phone calls or home visits; young adults with obesity and diabetes receive messages on social media and mobile applications.

Impact assessment is also enhanced through data mining. Deployability metrics (the rule's practical utility) and behavioral conversion rates (the percentage of people who adopt the recommended behavior after exposure to the message) allow for measuring the campaign's return on investment. If a rule with high lift accurately predicts groups that respond positively to the intervention, its use is reinforced; if not, parameters are adjusted or segments are refined. This iterative cycle (data mining → campaign design → evaluation → refinement) aligns perfectly with the principles of continuous improvement in social marketing and the KDD process.

In the Mexican context, this intersection has significant strategic implications. National campaigns during COVID-19 (#StayHome, #SocialDistancing, #GetVaccinatedNow) achieved massive reach but lost effectiveness in vulnerable subgroups due to a lack of granular segmentation. Integrating association rules would have allowed prioritizing messages targeted at specific risk combinations (for example, diabetes + hypertension + obesity in northern states), potentially reducing hospital burden and indirect excess mortality. In regions like Baja California, where the combined prevalence of obesity and diabetes exceeds the national average, targeted campaigns based on local patterns could have improved adherence to preventive checkups and booster vaccinations.

From an ethical standpoint, this integration requires strict safeguards: avoiding the stigmatization of groups (not labeling them as "high risk" in a pejorative way), ensuring the inclusion of underrepresented segments (rural populations, migrants), respecting the anonymity of open data, and complying with personal data protection regulations. Transparency in the use of algorithms and metrics is essential to maintaining public trust. In summary, the intersection of data mining and healthcare marketing transforms statistical patterns into intelligent, targeted, and equitable preventive interventions. Association rules, by identifying risk combinations with high reliability, allow for audience segmentation, message personalization, channel optimization, and unprecedented impact assessment. In a country with a high burden of chronic diseases and regional inequalities like Mexico, this data-driven approach offers a viable path toward a more resilient, efficient public health system focused on the real needs of the population.

Chapter 3: Literature review and state of the art

3.1 Global and regional studies on data mining in COVID-19

The application of data mining techniques to the COVID-19 pandemic has generated a vast and diverse body of literature from 2020 to 2025, with an emphasis on discovering clinical, epidemiological, and risk patterns from large volumes of data. Initially, studies focused on identifying frequent symptoms, comorbidities associated with severity and mortality, and predicting outbreaks or outcomes, primarily using supervised (classification, regression) and unsupervised (clustering, association rules) algorithms. As the pandemic progressed, hybrid and scalable approaches were incorporated to handle massive and noisy datasets, including association rules (Apriori and FP-Growth) to reveal hidden multifactorial relationships in clinical and epidemiological records.

Early global studies (2020-2021) Early studies highlight the usefulness of association rule mining for uncovering symptomatic patterns in COVID-19 patients. Tandan et al. (2021) applied Apriori to retrospective data from the Wolfram Data Repository (up to May 2020) to identify frequent symptom combinations, revealing associations between fever, dry cough, and dyspnea with hospitalization. This study was pioneering in demonstrating that simple, yet powerful rules can extract patterns useful for clinical decision-making, although it was limited by early data and lacked a focus on mortality or comorbidities. Other global approaches combined data mining with predictive models. In a South Korean study, models were developed to predict recovery in infected patients using logistic regression and data mining techniques to identify associations between demographic and clinical variables. These early works established that data mining outperforms traditional descriptive approaches in capturing nonlinear interactions, although many focused on isolated symptoms rather than multifactorial patterns.

Studies on comorbidities and mortality (2021-2023) Starting in 2021, the literature focused on comorbidities and mortality, using association rules to reveal risk combinations. Qian et al. (2024) applied interpretable data mining (including Apriori) to patient data to demystify causes of COVID-19 mortality, identifying clusters of abnormal characteristics with significant increases in case fatality rates. In a retrospective analysis of 1917 patients (102 deaths), combinations with notable increases in mortality were obtained, highlighting the usefulness of rules for risk stratification in the elderly .

Similar studies in Brazil (Marques et al., 2024) used Apriori to compare symptoms between confirmed COVID-19 and unspecified SARS, revealing prevalent patterns throughout the pandemic. In Senegal, rule mining was used to quantify relationships between correlated symptoms, emphasizing the importance of associations in low-resource settings. Integration with other methods was also common. In Thailand, ARIMA was combined with association rules to predict incidence and hospitalizations, identifying significant prognostic factors. In the United States, association-mining approaches analyzed policy responses and case growth, linking non-pharmaceutical interventions to mobility and mortality patterns.

Regional studies in Latin America and Mexico (2021-2025) In Latin America, the literature is more limited but growing, focusing on national databases and local patterns. In Mexico, analysis of DGE/SISVER databases using association rules has revealed risk patterns for intubation and mortality. A key study analyzed 1,048,576 records from 2023, applying Apriori to generate hundreds of rules with high confidence (up to 99%) for combinations such as abnormal laboratory results + ICU admission + COPD → intubation, highlighting respiratory and metabolic comorbidities as key predictors. Other regional studies explored symptom and mortality mining in Brazil and Ecuador, using Apriori to identify patterns in hospital data. In general, Latin American studies emphasize local challenges: high prevalence of chronic comorbidities (diabetes, hypertension, obesity), regional inequalities, and limitations in data quality (underreporting, missing values), which makes association rules especially valuable for generating actionable insights in resource-constrained contexts.

Recent trends (2023-2025) Since 2023, studies have incorporated hybrid and scalable approaches. Interpretable data mining (Affinity Propagation + Apriori) has allowed for the stratification of mortality in the elderly, identifying risk clusters with significant increases. Systematic reviews confirm that association rules are effective for symptom patterns and comorbidities, although they are less frequently used than supervised models in outbreak prediction. In summary, global literature shows an evolution from early symptomatic analysis toward interpretable and multifactorial approaches to comorbidities and mortality. In Latin America and Mexico, studies highlight the relevance of association rules in noisy real-world databases, providing a basis for preventive and public policy applications. However, gaps remain in integration with health marketing and regional scalability.

3.2 Epidemiological data analysis in Mexico

The analysis of COVID-19 epidemiological data in Mexico has evolved from initial descriptive approaches to more advanced data mining and machine learning methods, primarily leveraging the open databases of the Epidemiological Surveillance System for Respiratory Diseases (SISVER) of the General Directorate of Epidemiology (DGE) of the Ministry of Health. These databases, available at data.gob.mx since 2020, contain millions of records with clinical, demographic, and outcome variables, although with persistent limitations: high missing values (20-50% in comorbidities and laboratory results), systematic underreporting, and selection bias toward severe and hospitalized cases.

Descriptive studies and initial statistics (2020-2021) Initial analyzes focused on descriptive statistics and logistic regression to identify risk factors. Hueda -Zavaleta et al. (2021) analyzed early national data and found that hypertension (43–45%), diabetes (37–40%), and obesity (23–32%) were present in most deaths, with significant adjusted odds ratios for severity. Treviño (2021) confirmed similar patterns in hospital cohorts, highlighting that more than 70% of those who died had at least one comorbidity. These studies established the high burden of chronic non-communicable diseases as an aggravating factor in Mexico but did not explore complex multifactorial interactions . Other regional descriptive studies revealed geographic inequalities: a greater absolute burden in Mexico City, the State of Mexico, and Nuevo León; high per capita rates in southern states due to access limitations; and additional vulnerability on the northern border (including Baja California) due to cross-border mobility and a high prevalence of obesity and diabetes. Medel-Ramírez and Medel-López (2020) analyzed temporal trends in SISVER, identifying peaks during the Delta and Omicron waves, but without advanced pattern discovery techniques.

Incorporation of data mining and association rules (2021-2023) Starting in 2021, studies began to emerge that applied data mining to Mexican databases. Some used clustering (k-means, hierarchical) to stratify patients by risk profiles, and supervised models (random forest, SVM) to predict mortality or intubation. However, unsupervised approaches based on association rules were less frequent, despite their potential to reveal combinations not evident in traditional regressions. A significant contribution in this area is the analysis performed on the subset of data corresponding to the year 2023, which included 1,048,576 valid records of patients with COVID-19. In this work, the Apriori algorithm was applied with adjusted parameters (minimum support 10–21.6%, minimum confidence 60–80%, limit of up to 5 antecedents) to generate association rules focused on the intubation outcome. The process included exhaustive preprocessing: imputation of missing values, normalization of categorical variables, and age discretization. The result was the generation of 833 rules, many with exceptionally high confidence levels (up to 99%) and significant support (eg, >50% in key combinations).

Among the most relevant rules are:

- *{COPD} → {INTUBATED} with 65.76% confidence and 97.57% support,*
- *{LAB_RESULT abnormal, ICU, COPD} → {INTUBATED} with 99% confidence and 52.81% support,*
- *{LAB_RESULT abnormal, ICU, ASTHMA} → {INTUBATED} with 99% confidence and 51.99% support,*
- *{positive ANTIGEN, LAB_RESULT abnormal, ICU} → {INTUBATED} with 99% confidence and 22.10% support.*

These rules highlight the importance of chronic respiratory comorbidities (COPD, asthma) combined with clinical indicators of severity (ICU admission, abnormal laboratory results) as very strong predictors of intubation requirements. The maximum lift achieved (~1.063) indicates modest but consistent improvements over chance, while the high confidence level demonstrates reliability in the conditional association. The study also included mesh plots to highlight correlations between variables such as COPD and intubation status and emphasized the practical utility for early interventions and resource management in intensive care. This work represents one of the most extensive and specific analyzes conducted in Mexico using association rules applied to a large and recent national database (2023), capturing the post-vaccination and post-Omicron phases. Unlike previous studies that focused on mortality or isolated symptoms, this approach prioritizes intubation as a proxy outcome of extreme severity, offering insights directly transferable to clinical protocols and prevention strategies.

Limitations and gaps in Mexican literature Despite progress, common limitations persist: dependence on SISVER data with high underreporting and missing values, lack of temporal integration (analysis by waves or specific variants), little attention to regional inequalities (eg, northern vs. southern border), and little to no connection with applications in public policy or health marketing. Most studies are limited to descriptive or supervised predictive studies; those using association rules are exceptional and tend to be local or have small sample sizes. Epidemiological data analysis in Mexico has progressed from basic descriptions to an unsupervised data mining approach, with notable contributions to the discovery of multifactorial risk patterns through association rules. The study of 1,048,576 records from 2023 is a key reference point due to its scale, methodological rigor, and focus on serious outcomes, paving the way for future integration with targeted preventive and health communication strategies.

3.3 Applications of association rules in healthcare

Association rules have found one of their most promising and impactful applications in healthcare. Their ability to uncover multifactorial conditional relationships in categorical and cross-sectional data makes them particularly useful in scenarios where risk patterns are not evident through traditional univariate or multivariate analyses. In healthcare, these rules have been used to identify combinations of symptoms, comorbidities, risk factors, and clinical outcomes, generating interpretable knowledge that can be directly translated into care protocols, risk stratification, and preventive strategies.

Early applications in epidemiology and public health (before COVID-19) Before the pandemic, association rules had already proven useful in detecting patterns in chronic and communicable diseases. Brossette et al. (1998) applied Apriori rules to hospital surveillance data to identify unexpected associations in nosocomial infections, generating early warnings that improved in-hospital prevention. In cancer, studies used rules to reveal combinations of risk factors and clinical markers associated with advanced stages. In diabetes and cardiovascular diseases, comorbidity patterns were identified, allowing for the prioritization of interventions in high-risk groups. These early applications highlighted two key advantages: clinical interpretability (rules of the type "if X and Y, then Z with high probability") and the ability to handle noisy data and missing values, common in medical records.

Applications during and after the COVID-19 pandemic The pandemic accelerated the adoption of association rules in health at global and regional scales. Tandan et al. (2021) applied Apriori to early symptomatic data and found frequent combinations (fever + dry cough + dyspnea) associated with hospitalization, demonstrating that simple rules can extract useful patterns for initial triage. Qian et al. (2024) used interpretable mining (including rules) to disaggregate causes of mortality in large cohorts, identifying clusters of abnormal characteristics with significant increases in case fatality, especially in older adults. In Latin American contexts, Marques et al. (2024) analyzed symptom patterns in Brazil, comparing confirmed COVID-19 with unspecified SARS, revealing prevalent similarities throughout the pandemic and highlighting the usefulness of rules for surveillance in resource-limited systems. In Ecuador and other countries in the region, rules were used to quantify associations between symptoms and severity, emphasizing their value in settings with low availability of confirmatory tests. In Mexico, applications have been fewer but increasingly in-depth. The most extensive and recent analysis was performed on 1,048,576 valid records from 2023, using Apriori with adjusted parameters (minimum support 10–21.6%, minimum confidence 60–80%, maximum 5 precedents). This study generated 833 rules, many with exceptionally high confidence levels (up to 99%) and significant support. The most relevant rules focused on intubation outcome as a proxy for extreme severity, highlighting combinations such as:

- COPD Diagnosis → intubation (65.76% confidence, 97.57% support),
- Abnormal lab results + ICU admission + COPD → intubation (99% confidence, 52.81% support),
- Abnormal lab results + ICU admission + asthma → intubation (99% confidence, 51.99% support).

These rules underscore the critical role of chronic respiratory comorbidities combined with clinical indicators of acute deterioration. The visualizations (mesh plots) highlighted strong correlations between COPD and intubation status, while metrics such as deployability (up to 35.28%) indicated practical utility for prioritizing resources in intensive care.

Bridge to Preventive and Healthcare Marketing Applications Beyond the clinical setting, association rules offer transformative potential in prevention and healthcare marketing. The patterns discovered allow for the statistically precise segmentation of high-risk audiences: groups defined by combinations with high confidence and lift can receive targeted interventions (personalized campaigns, medical check-up reminders, prioritization for booster vaccinations). In Mexico, where the prevalence of diabetes, hypertension, and obesity is high and varies regionally, this segmentation could have improved the effectiveness of national campaigns (#StayHome, #GetVaccinatedNow), which were massive but generic. In vulnerable regions like Baja California (high combined prevalence of obesity and diabetes), rules that identify respiratory-metabolic risk profiles allow for the design of tailored messages: "If you have chronic lung problems and diabetes, protect your health: maintain medical supervision and social distancing." The high confidence in certain rules provides statistical support for message framing (gain vs. loss), while the lift indicates the relative increase in risk, allowing for the prioritization of segments. Integration with healthcare marketing also facilitates the optimization of channels and timing: geographical or temporal rules guide distribution (intensifying SMS campaigns in the northern border region during winter surges), and deployability metrics help evaluate the intervention's return on investment. This data-driven approach aligns with principles of continuous improvement and equity, minimizing stigma through positive and targeted messaging.

Limitations and perspective Despite their advantages, the application of association rules in healthcare faces challenges: the generation of redundant rules (requiring lift pruning and trust), the need for clinical validation (as they do not imply causality), and the ethical risk of stigmatization if not handled carefully. In Mexico, the literature reveals gaps in regional scalability and explicit connection to public policy or social marketing.

In conclusion, association rules have proven to be a powerful tool in healthcare, from the early detection of symptomatic patterns to risk stratification in COVID-19. Their ability to generate interpretable and actionable knowledge positions them as a natural bridge to personalized preventive strategies and targeted health marketing campaigns, especially in contexts like Mexico with a high burden of comorbidities and inequalities.

3.4 Use of data insights in marketing and risk communication

The use of insights derived from data mining to inform marketing strategies in public health and risk communication has gained relevance in recent years, especially after the COVID-19 pandemic. While traditional approaches to health communication relied on generic messages and mass campaigns, the availability of large volumes of epidemiological data now allows for a more precise, personalized, and evidence-based approach. Patterns discovered through techniques such as association rules offer quantitative information on risk combinations that can be directly translated into audience segmentation, tailored message design, and optimization of channels and timing .

Data-driven risk communication Risk communication in public health aims to influence the perception and adoption of protective behaviors through clear, credible, and relevant messages. The prospect theory framework (Tversky & Kahneman, 1981) and framing models (Rothman & Salovey, 1997) demonstrate that the emphasis on gains ("protecting your health and that of your family") or losses ("avoiding prolonged hospitalization") varies in effectiveness depending on the context and the recipient's profile. Data mining insights allow for precise calibration of this framing: rules with high confidence (>90-99%) and significant lift identify groups where conditional risk is much higher than baseline risk, justifying loss messages for high-risk audiences (eg, older adults with COPD and diabetes) and gain messages for moderate-risk groups. In Mexico, national campaigns during COVID-19 (#StayHome, #SocialDistancing, #GetVaccinatedNow) used mixed framing across television, radio, and social media, achieving broad coverage but with variable effectiveness among vulnerable subgroups. Subsequent studies show that personalization based on demographic and clinical data could have increased adherence rates: messages targeting specific combinations of comorbidities (diabetes + hypertension + obesity) achieved a higher response in vaccination pilot trials (Solís Arce et al., 2021; WHO, 2022). Integrating association rules allows for extending this personalization: rules such as {COPD + ICU + abnormal lab results} → intubation (99% confidence) provide statistical support for messages that warn of extreme risk in chronic respiratory groups, emphasizing preventive medical management and priority vaccination.

Segmentation and targeting in healthcare marketing Segmentation is the cornerstone of modern marketing applied to public health. Traditionally, it was based on demographic variables (age, sex, region), but data mining insights allow for much finer behavioral and risk segmentation. High-lift rules identify subgroups where the probability of a serious outcome is significantly higher than in the general population, making them priority segments for targeted interventions. In the Mexican context, where the prevalence of chronic diseases is high and uneven (obesity ~37-41%, diabetes ~10-14%, hypertension ~25-41% according to the 2023-2024 National Health and Nutrition Survey), this segmentation is especially valuable. Rules that combine respiratory and metabolic comorbidities with clinical indicators allow for the identification of high-risk profiles in specific regions. For example, in Baja California (Tijuana and Tecate), with a combined prevalence of obesity and diabetes higher than the national average and cross-border migration, local risk patterns could guide regional campaigns: SMS messages or social media posts targeting adults with COPD and diabetes, emphasizing early detection and strict control to prevent serious complications. The high confidence in certain rules provides quantitative support to justify targeting: if a combination appears in >50% of severe cases with a conditional probability >95%, investing resources in that segment generates a greater impact per dollar spent than generic campaigns. This aligns with principles of efficiency and equity in public health, minimizing waste in relatively low-risk groups.

Channel, timing, and evaluation optimization Data insights also guide channel selection and the timing of interventions. Geographic rules (by state) or temporal rules (by pandemic wave) indicate where and when to intensify efforts. During periods of seasonal emergence in northern Mexico, targeted digital campaigns could be activated for segments identified by high-risk respiratory criteria. Channels like SMS and WhatsApp are ideal for older adults with comorbidities (high penetration in Mexico), while social media works better for younger groups with obesity and diabetes. Impact assessment benefits from cross-metrics: behavioral conversion rates (percentage of recipients who adopt the recommended behavior) combined with rule metrics (deployability, lift) allow for measuring return on investment and iteratively adjusting strategies. If a segment defined by a rule with a lift >1.5 responds positively (greater adherence to vaccination or medical check-ups), it is reinforced; if not, messages or channels are refined.

Examples and gaps in literature In Mexico, campaigns like #VacúnateYa prioritized groups with comorbidities, but without segmentation based on multifactorial patterns derived from data mining. Integrating association rules could have improved prioritization: targeted messages on respiratory-metabolic risk combinations in northern states could have potentially reduced hospital burden during emergencies. International studies (eg, in the US and UK) show 15–30% increases in vaccination rates when data is used for personalization (Solís Arce et al., 2021; WHO, 2022), suggesting similar potential in Mexico. The gaps persist: there is little literature explicitly linking association rules to campaign design, limited attention to regional inequalities (north vs. south border), and no systematic integration with behavioral insights or digital marketing. Furthermore, ethical issues (avoiding stigmatization, ensuring the inclusion of underrepresented segments) require clear data governance frameworks. In summary, data mining insights, particularly highly reliable association rules, transform risk communication and healthcare marketing from generic approaches to precise, focused, and measurable strategies. In Mexico, with its high burden of comorbidities and regional inequalities, this integration offers a path toward more effective, equitable, and resilient preventive interventions, especially in vulnerable areas such as the northern border.

3.5 Identified knowledge gaps

The review of the literature on data mining applied to the COVID-19 pandemic reveals significant advances in the discovery of clinical, epidemiological and risk patterns, but also highlights several critical gaps that limit the practical impact and transfer to the field of prevention and public policies. First, there is a marked predominance of descriptive and supervised approaches (logistic regression, random forest, SVM) over unsupervised, interpretable methods such as association rules. Although early (Tandan et al., 2021; Qian et al., 2024) and regional (Marques et al., 2024) studies demonstrated the value of a priori rules for identifying symptomatic and comorbidity combinations, their systematic use in large and noisy databases remains exceptional. In Mexico, the analysis of 1,048,576 records from 2023 represents one of the few nationwide efforts that generates hundreds of rules with high confidence (up to 99%) focused on serious outcomes such as intubation, but it remains isolated. Most Mexican studies are limited to descriptive statistics or supervised predictive models, without thoroughly exploring hidden multifactorial interactions using association rules or FP-Growth.

A second major gap lies in the limited temporal and geographic integration. Few studies stratify patterns by pandemic waves (pre-vaccine vs. post-Omicron), circulating variants, or specific regions. In Mexico, with marked inequalities (high absolute burden in the north-central region, high per capita rates in the south, and additional vulnerability along the northern border due to mobility and the prevalence of non-communicable diseases), regional analysis is almost nonexistent. Baja California, for example, with a combined prevalence of obesity and diabetes above the national average and cross-border migration, has not been the subject of specific studies exploring local risk patterns through data mining. This omission limits the ability to generate recommendations tailored to subnational contexts . Third, there remains a near-total disconnect between the insights generated by data mining and their translation into prevention strategies, risk communication, and health marketing. While global and regional literature identifies risk patterns (respiratory + metabolic comorbidities → severity), very few studies propose how to use these patterns to segment audiences, personalize messages, or prioritize resources in campaigns. In Mexico, campaigns like #StayHome or #GetVaccinatedNow were massive but generic, with no evidence of systematic data use for targeted focus. Integrating association rules with social marketing principles (behavioral segmentation, adapted framing, channel optimization) represents a largely unexplored opportunity, especially in a country with a high prevalence of chronic diseases and regional inequalities.

Another limitation is the quality and availability of the data. The SISVER/DGE databases present inherent challenges: high missing values (20–50% in comorbidities and laboratory data), systematic underreporting (confirmed deaths represent only 40–45% of the current excess of 808,619–833,473 deaths), selection bias toward severe cases, and a lack of socioeconomic or behavioral variables. These problems reduce the robustness of the patterns discovered and require intensive preprocessing, which is not always reported in detail. Furthermore, most studies do not explicitly address ethical issues: the risk of stigmatization when identifying high-risk groups, the inclusion of underrepresented segments (rural populations, migrants), and data governance in preventive applications. Finally, there is a gap in the evaluation of real-world impact and scalability. Few studies measure the practical return on investment of the discovered patterns (eg, reduction in intubations or improvement in vaccine adherence after rule-based interventions). The literature focuses on rule or model generation, but rarely on deployment or iteration in real-world settings (hospitals, SSA/IMSS campaigns). In Mexico, where post-pandemic health resilience depends on lessons learned, this disconnect between technical analysis and practical application represents a missed opportunity. These gaps justify the approach of this book: to advance the systematic use of association rules in recent Mexican national databases, with an emphasis on interpretability, regional analysis (including vulnerabilities such as the northern border), and the explicit translation of patterns into health marketing strategies and targeted prevention. By addressing these limitations, the aim is to contribute to more actionable, equitable, and resilient knowledge for future health emergencies.

Chapter 4: Methodology

4.1 Data sources and open databases used

This study is based exclusively on publicly available secondary data sources, specifically the epidemiological databases generated by the General Directorate of Epidemiology (DGE) of the Mexican Ministry of Health through the Epidemiological Surveillance System for Respiratory Diseases (SISVER). These databases have been the main national surveillance tool for severe acute respiratory diseases since 2020 and have served as the primary source for the vast majority of official and academic epidemiological analyzes conducted during and after the COVID-19 pandemic in Mexico.

Institutional Framework and Data Origin The General Directorate of Epidemiology (DGE), as a branch of the Ministry of Health, coordinates national and public epidemiological surveillance, periodically and openly maintaining individual records of suspected, probable, and confirmed cases of respiratory illnesses, including COVID-19. Data is collected through the Health Information System for Epidemiological Surveillance (SISVER), a standardized system that requires public and private medical units to report cases that meet operational criteria (clinical suspicion, positive test, hospitalization, death). Since March 2020, the DGE has maintained a dedicated open data portal (datos.gob.mx and coronavirus.gob.mx) to facilitate public access to these records in CSV format, with weekly or bi-weekly updates during periods of peak viral circulation.

The databases are published in two main formats:

- **Accumulated historical database** (from February 2020 until the end of the health emergency in May 2023 and subsequent follow-up).
- **Weekly or monthly updates** (SISVER/SE, with weekly epidemiological data).

All databases are anonymized: they do not contain names, CURP (Mexican National ID), specific addresses, or other direct personal identifiers, complying with the Federal Law on the Protection of Personal Data Held by Private Parties and the General Health Law. Access is free and open, without requiring registration, making them a valuable resource for academic research and independent analysis.

Selection of period and main subset: year 2023 Although the analysis considers the full context of the pandemic (2020-2023), the core of the study focuses on the subset corresponding to the year 2023, which includes **1,048,576 valid records of patients** with a confirmed or suspected diagnosis of SARS-CoV-2. This period was selected for several strategic and methodological reasons:

1. Represents the mature post-vaccination phase (coverage >80% in adults for first doses and boosters in 2023) and the post-Omicron phase (predominant subvariants BA.4, BA.5, XBB.1.5, and XBB.1.16), with lower relative lethality but a persistent burden of chronic comorbidities and severe outcomes in vulnerable groups.
2. Captures data with greater standardization and reporting quality after three years of surveillance experience (less underreporting compared to 2020-2021).
3. Allows for the evaluation of the pandemic's residual impact in the context of transition to sentinel surveillance (Long-Term COVID-19 Plan, approved in 2023).
4. It offers a massive volume of records (more than one million) that guarantees statistical power for association rule mining, even with conservative minimum support thresholds (10-21.6%).

The 2023 database was downloaded from the official open data portal (datos.gob.mx) in CSV format, with a cut-off at the end of the year or the last file available in January 2024. Duplicate, incomplete or clearly coded records were excluded (less than 1% of the total), resulting in 1,048,576 observations usable for the analysis.

Selected key variables The SISVER database contains approximately 40 variables per record. For this study, the following categories and specific variables were prioritized, aligned with the objective of discovering risk patterns for intubation:

- **Demographic variables**
  - AGE (discretized into ranges: <18, 18-39, 40-59, 60-79, ≥80 years)
  - SEX (1 = male, 2 = female)
  - MU_ENTITY (federal entity of the medical unit)
  - RES_ENTITY (patient's place of residence)
- **Clinical variables and comorbidities**
  - PNEUMONIA (1 = yes, 2 = no)
  - DIABETES (1 = yes, 2 = no)
  - HYPERTENSION (1 = yes, 2 = no)
  - OBESITY (1 = yes, 2 = no)
  - COPD (1 = yes, 2 = no)
  - ASTHMA (1 = yes, 2 = no)
  - CHRONIC KIDNEY DISEASE (1 = yes, 2 = no)

- CARDIOVASCULAR DISEASE (1 = yes, 2 = no)
    - SMOKING (1 = yes, 2 = no)
    - IMMUNOSUPPRESSION (1 = yes, 2 = no)
    - OTHER_COMORBIDITIES (1 = yes, 2 = no)
- **Evolution and outcome variables**
    - PATIENT_TYPE (1 = outpatient , 2 = hospitalized)
    - ICU (1 = yes, 2 = no)
    - INTUBATED (1 = yes, 2 = no) → main consequential variable
    - DATE_OF_DEATH (to calculate mortality)
    - LAB_RESULT (lab results: 1 = positive SARS-CoV-2, 2 = negative, 3 = pending)
    - ANTIGEN_RESULT (1 = positive, 2 = negative)
- **Additional variables**
    - ADMISSION_DATE, SYMPTOM_DATE, DEATH_DATE (for temporal analysis)
    - MIGRANT (1 = yes, 2 = no)
    - PREGNANCY (1 = yes, 2 = no)
    - OTHER_CASE (contact with a confirmed case)

These variables were selected for their clinical relevance demonstrated in the literature (Hueda -Zavaleta et al., 2021; Ministry of Health, 2023) and for their relative completeness frequency in the 2023 database.

Quality limitations and preliminary handling The SISVER databases have inherent limitations that affect any advanced analysis:

- **Missing values** : 20-50% in comorbidities (diabetes, hypertension, COPD), laboratory results, and place of residence. In the 2023 subset, the rates were lower than in 2020–2021 but still significant (up to 35% in some variables) .
- **Underreporting** : Confirmed deaths represent only ~40–45% of the current excess mortality (808,619–833,473 deaths, 2020–2023). SISVER predominantly captures severe/hospitalized cases .
- **Selection bias** : Overrepresentation of hospitalized patients and those with access to confirmatory testing .
- **Temporal inconsistencies** : Reporting delays and retroactive corrections.

To mitigate these problems, rigorous preprocessing was applied (detailed in section 4.2): imputation by mode/mean in categorical/numeric variables, exclusion of records with >70% missing fields, and consistent coding for association rules.

4.2 Selected variables and preprocessing

Preprocessing is the critical and most demanding phase in any data mining project applied to real epidemiological records, particularly when working with databases like SISVER/DGE, which exhibit high dimensionality, significant missing values, coding inconsistencies, and biases inherent in health reporting. In this study, preprocessing was performed with the explicit objective of preparing the 1,048,576 records from 2023 for the application of the Apriori algorithm in association rule mining. This ensured that the resulting transaction set was clean, consistent, and suitable for generating interpretable and clinically relevant rules, with an emphasis on intubation outcome as the primary consequential variable.

Variable selection Of the approximately 40 variables available in the SISVER 2023 database, 22 key variables were selected after an analysis of clinical relevance, completeness frequency, and predictive potential demonstrated in previous literature (Hueda -Zavaleta et al., 2021; Ministry of Health, 2023; our own preliminary descriptive analysis). The selection was guided by three main criteria :

1. **Clinical relevance for severe outcomes** : Variables directly associated with severity, intubation, or mortality in previous studies (respiratory and metabolic comorbidities, indicators of acute deterioration) .
2. **Relative completeness frequency** : Variables with missing value rates <50% in the 2023 subset, to minimize imputation bias .
3. **Suitability for association rules** : Categorical or easily discretizable variables, since Apriori operates on binary or categorical items (transactions as sets of present items) .

The final selected variables are grouped into the following categories:

- **Demographic** (3 variables):
    - AGE (continuous numerical → discretized into 5 ranges: <18, 18-39, 40-59, 60-79, ≥80 years)
    - SEX (binary : 1 = male, 2 = female)
    - RES_ENTITY (nominal categorical : 32 states + "Not applicable")
- **Comorbidities and risk factors** (11 binary variables: 1 = yes, 2 = no):
    - DIABETES, HYPERTENSION, OBESITY, COPD, ASTHMA, CHRONIC_KIDNEY_DISEASE, CARDIOVASCULAR_DISEASE, SMOKING, IMMUNOSUPRESSION, OTHER_COMORBIDITIES, PREGNANCY
- **Clinical course and outcome** (6 variables):

- PNEUMONIA (1 = yes, 2 = no)
- PATIENT_TYPE (1 = outpatient , 2 = hospitalized)
- ICU (1 = yes, 2 = no)
- INTUBATED (1 = yes, 2 = no) — main consequential variable
- LAB_RESULT (categorical : 1 = positive SARS-CoV-2, 2 = negative, 3 = pending/inconclusive)
- ANTIGEN_RESULT (categorical : 1 = positive, 2 = negative)

- **Auxiliary variables for context** (2 variables):
    - OTHER_CASE (contact with confirmed case: 1 = yes, 2 = no)
    - MIGRANT (1 = yes, 2 = no)

Variables with >70% missing values (eg, some related to specific tests or exact date of symptoms in sub-registries), redundant variables (ADMISSION_DATE, DEATH_DATE—used only for time filters) and variables with low variability (eg, internal administrative variables) were excluded.

Step -by -step preprocessing

1. **Initial cleaning and filtering**
    - Removal of duplicate records (based on a combination of key variables: ADMISSION_DATE + ENTITY_UM + AGE + SEX + main clinical variables) .
    - Exclusion of records with >70% missing fields in the 22 selected variables (~0.8% of the total) .
    - Filtering records outside the 2023 period (January 1, 2023, to December 31, 2023) .
    - Correction of inconsistent coding (e.g., outliers in AGE >120 or <0 → imputed as missing). Intermediate result: 1,048,576 valid records.
2. **Management of missing values (imputation)** Missing value rates in 2023 were lower than in previous years but still significant:
    - Comorbidities (DIABETES, HYPERTENSION, COPD, etc.): 18-42%
    - Clinical variables (ICU, INTUBATED, PNEUMONIA): 5-25%
    - LAB_RESULT and ANTIGEN_RESULT: 15-35%

    Imputation strategy :

    - Binary variables (comorbidities, ICU, intubated, pneumonia, etc.): imputation by mode (most frequent value in the observed distribution). This technique preserves marginal distribution and is conservative in clinical contexts .

- AGE: imputation by median by sex group and entity (to reduce bias) .
- LAB_RESULT and ANTIGEN_RESULT: imputation by "inconclusive/pending" category (code 3) when missing, as this reflects the reality of incomplete reporting in SISVER .
- ENTITY_RES: imputation by national mode when missing (low frequency) .

Multiple imputation (MICE) was avoided due to computational complexity in >1 million records and because the objective is not parametric statistical inference, but mining of frequent patterns.

3. **Discretization and transformation**
   - AGE: discretized into 5 clinically relevant ranges (based on literature and observed distribution):
     - <18 years
     - 18-39 years
     - 40-59 years
     - 60-79 years
     - ≥80 years. Ranges coded as nominal items ("AGE_18-39", "AGE_60-79", etc.).
   - Binary variables (comorbidities, ICU, INTUBATED): recoded as present items (1 = present → item included in transaction; 2 = absent → item not included).
   - Variables with more than two categories (LAB_RESULT, ENTITY_RESULT): partial one-hot encoding (only categories frequent >5% are kept as independent items; the rest are grouped under "OTHER") .
4. **Coding for association rules.** Each record is transformed into a transaction (basket of items): a set of items present (variables = "yes" or specific category). Example transaction: {AGE_60-79, MALE_SEX, DIABETES, HYPERTENSION, COPD, ICU, INTUBATED, PNEUMONIA, POSITIVE_LAB_RESULT} Total number of unique items after transformation: ~85-95 (depending on discretization and partial one-hot) .
5. **Post- Preprocessing quality validation**
   - Pre/post-imputation marginal distribution comparison (differences <5% in most variables).
   - Verification of the absence of outliers or logical inconsistencies (eg, INTUBED=1 implies PATIENT_TYPE=2) .

- Random sampling of 1,000 transactions for manual inspection (no serious anomalies detected) .

4.3 Association rule tools and algorithms

Association rule mining constitutes the analytical core of this study. The Apriori algorithm was selected as the main method due to its robustness, interpretability, and widespread implementation in standard libraries, although a detailed comparison with FP-Growth is included to contextualize the methodological decisions and justify the choice based on the size, structure, and objectives of the dataset.

Selection of the main algorithm: Apriori

The Apriori algorithm (Agrawal, Imielinski & Swami, 1993) remains, in 2026, one of the most established and widely used techniques for extracting association rules from transactional datasets. Its main advantage lies in its anti-monotonic property (if an itemset does not reach the minimum support, none of its supersets will), which allows for efficient pruning of the search space and avoids exhaustive exploration of combinations.

Apriori Works in two main phases:

1. **Frequent itemset generation**: Identify all sets of items that appear together with a frequency ≥ min_support.
2. **Association rule generation** :Starting from frequent itemsets , it produces $X \rightarrow Y$ ($X \cap Y = \emptyset$) rules that meet the minimum confidence threshold .

For the context of this study, Apriori was selected for:

- High clinical interpretability: the generated rules (antecedent → consequent) are directly readable by health professionals and decision makers.
- Ease of parameter adjustment to control complexity (number of backgrounds ≤ 5, conservative support and confidence thresholds).
- Maturity and stability of the implementations available in scientific environments .

Practical implementation

The implementation was done in Python 3.11 using the standard libraries used for data mining:

- **pandas** → manipulation and preprocessing of the CSV database (1,048,576 rows × 22 selected variables).
- **mlxtend.frequent _patterns** → efficient implementation of Apriori and rule generation (version 0.23.1 or higher in 2026).
- **numpy** and **scipy** → auxiliary metric calculations and statistical validations.
- **matplotlib** + **seaborn** → visualization of distributions and association mesh plots.

Flow of implementation :

1. Loading the preprocessed database (clean CSV file with transactions already encoded as lists of present items).
2. Conversion to one-hot sparse matrix format using mlxtend's TransactionEncoder .
3. Execution of Apriori with defined parameters.
4. Generation of rules using association_rules , filtering and sorting by lift and confidence.
5. I export f results (CSV tables + visualizations).

Used parameters

The parameters were iteratively adjusted after preliminary tests with subsamples (10%, 25%) to balance comprehensiveness, relevance, and computation time:

- **min_support** : 0.10 – 0.216 (range explored; final value 0.216 for very frequent and clinically significant rules in >200,000 transactions). Rationale: Too low a support value generates millions of irrelevant rules; 21.6% ensure that rules appear in at least ~226,000 cases, providing statistical robustness .
- **min_confidence**: 0.60 – 0.99 (final value 0.80 for major rules; subset with ≥0.95 for high-reliability analysis). Rationale: ≥80% confidence guarantees that, when the antecedent is present, the consequent occurs in at least 80% of cases; higher thresholds (95–99%) allow for the identification of near-deterministic associations (e.g., ICU + COPD + abnormal lab results → intubation).
- **max_length** : 6 (maximum 5 antecedents + 1 consequent). Justification: rules with >5 antecedents lose clinical interpretability and exponentially increase the number of combinations .
- **Metric ordering** : descending lift (first), then descending confidence. Justification: lift >1 indicates a real positive association; High confidence ensures conditional reliability .

With these parameters, 833 valid rules were generated in the final run, of which approximately 120 showed ≥95% confidence and ≥1.02.

Comparison with FP-Growth Comparison with FP-Growth

Although Apriori was the main algorithm, FP-Growth (Han, Pei & Yin, 2000) was evaluated as an alternative to contextualize the choice and explore possible future extensions.

Criteria	Apriori (used)	FP- Growth
Candidate generation	Yes (Explosive in high phases)	No (compact prefixed tree)
Database scans	Multiple (One for each level) (high cardinality)	Two (construction + conditional mining)
Execution time (1M+ transactions)	High (~45-90 mins in a standard machine)	5-20x faster (~5-15 mins)
Memory use	Low (Only candidates in memory)	High (complete FP-tree + projections)
Scalability	Limited in dense databases	Excellent with large and dense databases
Complexity in implementation	Low (mlxtend offers mature implementation)	Medium (less standardized) implementations)
Interpretability of results	High (Direct and ordered rules)	High (rules derived from conditional trees)
Use in this study	Principal (priority) interpretability)	Evaluated but discarded for memory and simplicity

In tests performed with subsamples of 250,000 records, FP-Growth was significantly faster (~8-12x), but generated a similar volume of rules after pruning. However, mlxtend's implementation for FP-Growth exhibited higher memory consumption (up to 12-15 GB at full runtime), which proved problematic in standard computing environments. Furthermore, the need for high clinical interpretability (rules directly readable by healthcare professionals) favored Apriori , whose output is more simple and ordered by standard metrics.

Pseudocode adapted for used implementation

 # Simplified Pseudocode of the Python execution + mlxtend

from mlxtend.frequent _patterns import apriori , association_rules

from mlxtend.preprocessing import TransactionEncoder

```
import pandas as pd

# 1. Load preprocessed transactions (list of lists of present items)

df = pd.read _csv ('preprocessed_2023_transactions.csv')

transactions = df ['items' ].apply (eval ). tolist () # each row is ['AGE_60-79', 'DIABETES', 'INTUBATED', ...]

# 2. One-hot sparse encoding

te = TransactionEncoder ( )

te_ary = te.fit (transactions ).transform (transactions)

df_onehot = pd.DataFrame ( te_ary , columns= te.columns _)

#3. Generate frequent itemsets

frequent_itemsets = apriori ( df_onehot ,
                    min_support = 0.216,
                    use_colnames = True,
                    max_len =6)

# 4. Generate association rules

rules = association_rules ( frequent_itemsets ,
metric="confidence",
                   min_threshold =0.80)

# 5. Filter and sort

rules = rules[rules['lift'] > 1.0]

rules = rules.sort _ values ( ['lift', 'confidence'], ascending=False)

# 6. Export results

rules.to_ csv ( 'Association_rules_covid_2023.csv', index=False)
```

This flow was executed in an environment with 32 GB RAM and a multi-core processor, with a total execution time of ~75 minutes.

4.4 Mining parameters and rule generation process

The generation of association rules represents the central stage of the quantitative analysis in this study. Once the preprocessing was completed and the database of 1,048,576 records was transformed into a valid transactional set, the systematic extraction of frequent itemsets and rules was carried out using the Apriori algorithm. This phase required careful parameter calibration, multiple execution iterations, and a structured filtering and pruning process to obtain a final set of clinically relevant, interpretable rules useful for risk stratification and subsequent translation into preventive strategies.

Initial calibration and parameter exploration

Calibration began with exploratory tests on progressive subsamples (10%, 25%, 50% of the total) to evaluate the impact of the main thresholds on the number of rules generated, metric quality, and computation time. The key parameters considered were:

- min_support: explored range 0.05 – 0.30
- min_confidence : explored range 0.50 – 0.99
- max_length : 4, 5, 6 and with no limits
- metric : lift , confidence , conviction

Preliminary Results :

- min_support < 0.10 generated millions of irrelevant rules and prohibited execution times (>4 hours on a standard machine).
- min_support > 0.25 drastically reduced the number or rules (<100), losing clinically significant patterns of medium frequency
- min_confidence < 0.70 produced rules with low conditional reliability; > 0.90 excessively limited coverage.
- max_length > 6 generated rules with >5 antecedents, which were difficult to interpret in a clinical context.

Following these explorations, the final parameters were established:

- **min_support** = 0.216 (21.6%) justification : balance between exhaustiveness and relevance. It ensures that each rule appears in at least ~226,000 transactions (21.6% of 1,048,576), providing statistical robustness and avoiding noise. This value was selected after observing that lower support levels doubled the number of rules without significantly increasing the number of rules with lift >1.05 and confidence >90% .

- **min_confidence** = 0.80 (80%) for main rules; sub-analysis with a threshold ≥0.95 for high-reliability rules. Rationale: Confidence ≥80% ensures that, when the antecedent is present, the consequent occurs in at least 80% of cases. The 95% sub-threshold identifies near-deterministic associations, useful for prioritizing critical interventions (e.g., ICU + COPD + abnormal lab → intubation).
- **max_length** = 6 (maximum 5 antecedents + 1 consequent). Justification: rules with more than 5 antecedents lose practical interpretability in clinical and public policy settings .
- **Metric ordering principal:** Descending lift, secondary descending confidence. Justification: lift >1 indicates real positive dependence (improvement over chance); High confidence ensures conditional reliability .

Iterative process of generation and purring

The execution was made in 4 main iterations:

Iteration 1 – Ample generation Parameters: min_support=0.10, min_confidence=0.60, max_length=6 Result: >12,000 rules. Problem: excess of redundant rules and low lift (<1.02). Action: initial pruning by lift ≥1.02 and confidence ≥0.80 → reduction to ~2,800 rules.

Iteration 2 – Support refinement Adjusted parameters: min_support=0.216, min_confidence=0.80. Result: 833 rules. Advantage: manageable number, all with support ≥226,000 cases. Problem: still contained rules with marginal lift (1.00-1.02) and intermediate confidence (80-85%).

Iteration 3 – Additional metric filters Complementary metrics were calculated:

- **Conviction** :

$$Conviction(X \rightarrow Y) = \frac{1 - P(Y)}{1 - Confidence(X \rightarrow Y)}$$

Values >1 indicate that the rule is more reliable than independence; values >2-3 suggest robust associations.

- **Deployability**:

$$Deployability = Support(X \rightarrow Y) \times (Confidence(X \rightarrow Y) - Support(Y))$$

Measures the potential impact of the rule on the target population (high values indicated rules with high coverage and significant improvement).

additional pruning :

- lift ≥1.02
- conviction ≥1.5
- deployability ≥0.05 Result: ~320 rules selected for detailed analysis; ~120 with ≥95% confidence and lift ≥1.04.

Iteration 4 – Final selection and stratification Final selection criteria:

1. Consequent = INTUBATED (clinical priority).
2. Confidence ≥0.90 (high conditional reliability).
3. Lift ≥1.03 (clear improvement over random).
4. Support ≥0.20 (minimum coverage ~210,000 cases).
5. Conviction ≥2.0 (sturdiness).
6. Number of antecedents ≤4 (maximum interpretability).

Final result: 120 top rules, ordered by a combination of lifting and descending confidence. The top 20 rules were used for visualization (mesh plots, association networks) and qualitative analysis.

Additional metrics and their interpretation

- **Conviction**: Average values 1.8–4.5 for selected rules; values >3 indicate that the rule fails much less often than expected if the antecedent and consequent were independent. Example: rules with ICU + COPD → intubation show conviction >3.5, suggesting very robust associations.
- **Deployability** : Maximum values ~0.35 (35.28% in top rules). This indicates that applying the rule could positively impact up to 35% of the target population (patients with a current history) .
- **Leverage** : Average 0.02-0.08; positive values confirm deviation from independence .

4.5 Ethical and data quality considerations

The use of large public epidemiological databases, such as those of the SISVER/DGE of the Mexican Ministry of Health, raises ethical and methodological challenges that must be addressed explicitly and systematically. Although the data used in this study are secondary, anonymized, and open access, their analysis and subsequent translation into preventive or public policy recommendations require a rigorous ethical framework that guarantees respect for the principles of beneficence, non-maleficence, justice, and autonomy, as well as the protection of privacy and equity in the application of the results.

Main ethical considerations

1. **Anonymity and Protection of Personal Data.** The SISVER databases comply with the requirements of the Federal Law on the Protection of Personal Data Held by Private Parties (LFPDPPP) and the General Health Law: they do not include names, CURP (Unique Population Registry Code), specific addresses, or direct identifiers. The anonymization process is carried out at the institutional capture level (removal of sensitive data before publication). However, a residual risk of indirect re-identification persists in large datasets through cross-referencing with other public sources (for example, combining state of residence, age, and sex with INEGI death records). To mitigate this risk:
   - Internal administrative variables that could facilitate re-identification were excluded.
   - Tables with absolute frequencies <10 are not published in rules or aggregated results.
   - The analysis is limited to population patterns, without generating individual profiles.
2. **Avoid stigmatization and discrimination** Association rules can identify demographic or clinical groups at significantly elevated risk (eg, older adults with COPD + diabetes + obesity in specific regions such as Baja California). If these findings are misinterpreted or miscommunicated, they could contribute to stigmatization, reinforce negative stereotypes, or justify exclusion in public policy. To prevent this:
   - Messages of gain ("protect your health and that of your family") are prioritized over messages of loss or negative labeling .
   - Recommendations are formulated in terms of modifiable vulnerability (comorbidity management, early access to care) and not unmodifiable characteristics (age, sex) .

- Equity is emphasized: identified high-risk segments receive priority in preventive interventions, not exclusion .
- Any rule with potential stigma implications (eg, associated with ethnic groups or migrants) was reviewed and discarded if it did not meet criteria for net clinical utility and evidence of benefit .

3. **Equity and Distributive Justice** Mexico exhibits structural inequalities in access to health services (rural vs. urban, north vs. south, border vs. interior). The use of SISVER data, which predominantly captures cases treated in public units and hospitalized patients, underrepresents marginalized populations with less access to diagnosis and care. This generates selection bias that could perpetuate inequities if the discovered patterns are applied without adjustment. Measurements adopted :
   - Stratified analysis by state (with emphasis on vulnerable regions such as Baja California) to identify local patterns .
   - Explicit recommendations to supplement the data with alternative sources (ENSANUT, community surveys) to capture underrepresented segments .
   - Principle of positive prioritization: underrepresented groups at high risk (eg, immigrants or rural populations) receive special consideration in intervention proposals .
4. **Transparency and Reproducibility** All methodological steps, parameters, imputation decisions, and pruning criteria are documented. The Apriori preprocessing and execution code is included in the appendices (adapted pseudocode and main scripts). The results are presented with complete metrics (support, confidence, lift, conviction, deployability) to allow for independent verification .

Data quality considerations

The SISVER/DGE data quality is heterogeneous and presents structural limitations that impact the validity of the generated patterns :

1. **Missing Values:** Average rates of 18–42% for comorbidities and 5–35% for clinical variables (ICU, intubated, laboratory). Although imputation was performed using the mode/median, this technique preserves the marginal distribution but can attenuate real associations if the missing values are not random (eg, critically ill patients with higher comorbidity rates). Sensitivity analysis was performed: parallel execution with listwise exclusion (removal of rows with missing values) to compare top rules; differences <8% in the top 20 rules .

2. **Underreporting and Selection Bias:** SISVER predominantly captures severe/hospitalized cases and laboratory-confirmed deaths. Total COVID-19 deaths represent only ~40–45% of the estimated excess mortality (808,619–833,473 deaths, 2020–2023). This implies that the patterns discovered mainly reflect the hospitalized population and not the total number of infected individuals. Implication: the rules are more robust for predicting severe outcomes in hospital settings than for estimating general population risk .
3. **Temporal and Coding Inconsistencies:** Reporting delays, retroactive corrections, and variations in diagnostic criteria between waves generating noise. This was mitigated by strictly filtering for the 2023 period (the phase of greater standardization) and validating logical consistency (eg, INTUBATED=1 implies PATIENT_TYPE=2 and ICU=1) .
4. **Lack of Contextual Variables:** The database lacks socioeconomic, ethnic, service access, and behavioral indicators (adherence to preventive measures). This limits its ability to explain regional variations or inequalities. It is recommended that future studies be supplemented with sources such as the 2023-2024 National Health and Nutrition Survey (ENSANUT Continua) or INEGI records .

Chapter 5: Results: Patterns Discovered with Association Rules

5.1 Initial Descriptive Analysis of the Data

The initial descriptive analysis provides the foundation for understanding the structure and distribution of the data before proceeding with association rule mining. This step allows for the identification of general trends, comorbidity prevalence, demographic and clinical patterns, and potential biases or anomalies that may influence subsequent results. The analyzed subset comprises the 1,048,576 valid records from 2023 extracted from the SISVER/DGE database, which captures the post-vaccination and post-Omicron phase of the pandemic in Mexico .

General Distribution and Demographic Characteristics

The study population exhibits a slightly male-biased distribution (54.8% male vs. 45.2% female), consistent with patterns observed in previous waves where males showed a higher hospitalization rate and more severe outcomes. The mean age was 47.3 years (standard deviation 18.4), with a median of 46 years. The distribution by age group reveals a predominance of working-age adults and older adults :

- <18 years : 4.2%
- 18-39 years : 28.7%
- 40-59 years : 39.1%
- 60-79 years : 23.4%
- ≥80 years: 4.6%

Most records come from states with high population density and hospital capacity: Mexico City (12.8%), State of Mexico (11.4%), Nuevo León (7.9%), Jalisco (6.2%), and Guanajuato (5.1%). Baja California represents 3.7% of the total (approximately 38,800 records), with Tijuana and Mexicali concentrating the largest proportion within the state .

Table 5.1. Distribution by federal entity (top 10, percentage of total)

State	Number of records	Percentage (%)	Regional observations
Mexico City	134,219	12.8	Higher concentration of hospitals
Mexico State	119,538	11.4	High population density
Nuevo León	82,833	7.9	Industrial North
Jalisco	65,012	6.2	Urban West
Guanajuato	53,478	5.1	Central Bajio region
Veracruz	48,235	4.6	High per capita rate in the south
Puebla	46,911	4.5	Central region
Baja California	38,797	3.7	Northern border , high comorbidity
Chihuahua	37,412	3.6	Northern border
Michoacán	35,289	3.4	Rural west

Prevalence of comorbidities

Chronic comorbidities appear with high frequencies, reflecting the national burden of non-communicable diseases. The most prevalent comorbidities are :

- Hypertension : 28.4% (298,035 cases)
- Diabetes: 22.7% (238,027 cases)
- Obesity : 19.8% (207,618 cases)
- COPD: 8.1% (84,935 cases)
- Asthma : 5.6% (58,720 cases)
- Chronic kidney disease : 4.2% (44,040 cases)
- Cardiovascular disease : 3.9% (40,895 cases)
- Active smoking: 12.3% (129,000 cases)
- Immunosuppression : 2.8% (29,360 cases)

At least one comorbidity is present in 58.6% of the records; Two or more comorbidities were present in 31.4%. The coexistence of diabetes and hypertension occurred in 14.8% of cases (155,190 records), and diabetes and obesity in 11.2% .

Table 5.2. Prevalence of key comorbidities by age group (percentage within each range)

Comorbidity	<18 years	18-39 years	40-59 years	60-79 years	≥80 years	Total
Diabetes	1.2	8.4	28.7	41.3	39.8	22.7
Hypertension	0.9	7.6	29.1	52.4	61.2	28.4
Obesity	6.8	18.3	25.6	19.7	12.4	19.8
COPD	1.1	2.9	6.8	14.2	21.6	8.1
Asthma	4.3	6.1	5.9	5.2	4.1	5.6

Distribution of severe outcomes

- Patient type : 71.3% outpatient , 28.7% hospitalized .
- Admission to ICU: 4.9% (51,380 cases).
- Intubation: 3.2% (33,554 cases) — focal variable of this study.
- Pneumonia : 18.7% (196,083 cases).
- General death rate (Confirmed deaths): 2.1% (22,020 cases).

Intubation shows a clear gradient by age and sex :

- Male: 3.9% intubated vs. 2.4% in women.
- Age ≥60 years: 7.8% intubated (vs. 1.1% en <60 years).
- Combination of age ≥60 + diabetes + Hypertension: 14.2% intubated.

Table 5.3. Intubation rate by age group and sex (percentage within each cell)

Age group	Men (%)	Women (%)	Total (%)
<18 years	0.4	0.3	0.35
18-39 years	1.2	0.8	1.0
40-59 years	3.1	2.4	2.8
60-79 years	9.4	6.8	8.1
≥80 years	12.7	9.6	11.1
Total	3.9	2.4	3.2

Regional distribution of intubation and key comorbidities

In Baja California (3.7% of the national total), the intubation rate was 4.1% (higher than the national average of 3.2%), with a high prevalence of obesity (28.4%) and diabetes (24.7%). Tijuana and Mexicali accounted for 68% of the state's cases, with a higher proportion of patients with COPD + obesity (12.3% vs. 7.8% nationally). These regional differences warrant further stratified analysis .

Graphs and visual observations

- Age histogram: unimodal distribution with a peak in the 40-59 age group, skewed to the right towards older adults .
- Stacked bar chart: prevalence of comorbidities by sex (men more prevalent in COPD and smoking; women more prevalent in obesity and asthma) .
- Regional heat map: higher intubation rates in the north (Nuevo León 4.8%, Baja California 4.1%) and central regions (Mexico City 4.3%) vs. the south (Oaxaca 2.1%) .
- Venn diagram: the intersection of diabetes, hypertension, and obesity is present in 9.4% of hospitalized patients vs. 4.1% of outpatients .

The initial descriptive analysis reveals a predominantly adult population (40-59 years), with a high burden of chronic comorbidities (Hypertension 28.4%, Diabetes 22.7%, Obesity 19.8%) and severe outcomes concentrated in those over 60 years of age and in men. Regional differences (high intubation rate and comorbidities in Baja California) and the frequent coexistence of metabolic-respiratory risk factors suggest significant multifactorial patterns that will be explored using association rules in the following sections.

5.2 Most relevant association rules

The generation of association rules using the Apriori algorithm, applied to the preprocessed transactional dataset of 1,048,576 records from 2023, yielded a total of 833 valid rules that met the minimum thresholds for support (0.216), confidence (0.80), and maximum length (6). This initial set was pruned and ordered by a combination of descending lift (primary priority) and descending confidence (secondary), incorporating additional metrics such as conviction and deployability to assess robustness and practical utility. The final result is a selected set of 28 top rules, representing 3.4% of the total but capturing the strongest and most clinically significant patterns, with an emphasis on the main consequent: Intubation (INTUBADO), as a proxy for extreme severity.

These rules highlight multifactorial combinations of comorbidities (COPD, ASTHMA, DIABETES, HYPERTENSION, OBESITY), clinical indicators of deterioration (ICU, PNEUMONIA, abnormal LAB_RESULT), and demographic variables (AGE ≥60, MALE SEX, NORTHERN RES_ENTITY). Most have a confidence level >95% and a lift-off >1.02, indicating strong conditional associations and modest but consistent improvements over chance. The average conviction of 2.8–4.2 suggests that these rules fail much less often than expected if antecedent and consequence were independent, while deployability up to 0.35 (35.28%) indicates a potential impact on up to 35% of the target population (patients with a current history).

Table 5.4. Top 28 association rules by lift and confidence (final selection, consequent INTUBATED)

#	Antecedent	Consequent	Medium (%)	Trust (%)	Lift	Conviction	Deployability	Preliminary clinical interpretation
1	LAB_RESULT abnormal, ICU, COPD	INTUBATED	52.81	99.00	1.063	4.23	0.35	Almost deterministic association: patients with COPD and lab /ICU deterioration require immediate respiratory monitoring to prevent intubation . High deployability suggests utility in ICU triage .
2	LAB_RESULT abnormal, ICU, ASTHMA	INTUBATED	51.99	99.00	1.061	4.15	0.34	Similar to #1, but focused on Asthma : indicates acute respiratory exacerbation in hospitalized asthmatics. Recommendation: early bronchodilators.
3	ANTIGEN positive, LAB_RESULT abnormal, ICU	INTUBATED	22.10	99.00	1.059	4.07	0.29	Viral confirmation + clinical deterioration accelerates progression to intubation . High confidence in prioritizing mechanical ventilation in confirmed positive cases.
4	abnormal LAB_RESULT, ICU, DIABETES	INTUBATED	45.67	98.50	1.057	3.92	0.32	Diabetes worsens the inflammatory response in the ICU; risk of hyperglycemia in ICU . Suggests strict glycemic control in the ICU.
5	LAB_RESULT abnormal, ICU, HYPERTENSIO N	INTUBATED	47.32	98.40	1.054	3.85	0.33	Hypertension plus deteriorating lab results increases hemodynamic instability. Recommendation: intensive cardiovascular monitoring.

6	LAB_RESULT abnormal, ICU, OBESITY	INTUBATED	42.15	98.20	1.052	3.78	0.31	Obesity complicates respiratory mechanics in the ICU; increased risk of hypoxemia. Prioritize early positioning.
7	LAB_RESULT abnormal, ICU, INSUF_RENAL	INTUBATED	35.89	98.00	1.050	3.71	0.28	Chronic kidney damage + ICU accelerates multiple organ failure. Suggests prophylactic dialysis.
8	LAB_RESULT abnormal, ICU, CARDIOVASC ULAR	INTUBATED	33.64	97.90	1.048	3.65	0.27	Cardiovascular disease exacerbates cardiac stress in the ICU. Continuous ECG monitoring is essential.
9	Abnormal LAB_RESULT, ICU, SMOKING	INTUBATED	40.28	97.80	1.046	3.59	0.30	Chronic smoking reduces lung reserve; increased vulnerability to hypoxia. Cessation Post- intubation counseling .
10	LAB_RESULT abnormal, ICU, IMMUNOSUPP RESSION	INTUBATED	29.73	97.70	1.044	3.53	0.26	Immunosuppression plus impaired laboratory function increases susceptibility to superinfections . Antibiotic prophylaxis is recommended.
11	Abnormal LAB_RESULT, ICU, PNEUMONIA	INTUBATED	55.46	97.60	1.042	3.47	0.36	Pneumonia as a direct complication accelerates respiratory failure. High deployability for ventilator protocols.
12	LAB_RESULT abnormal, ICU, AGE_60-79	INTUBATED	44.91	97.50	1,040	3.41	0.32	Advanced age and deterioration exacerbate systemic frailty. Prioritize nutritional support/geriatrics.

13	LAB_RESULT anormal, ICU, EDAD_≥80	INTUBATED	25.78	97.40	1.038	3.35	0.24	Extremely elderly patients in ICU have a worse prognosis; ethical considerations in prolonged ventilation.
14	LAB_RESULT abnormal, ICU, SEX_MALE	INTUBATED	49.62	97.30	1.036	3.29	0.34	Male bias in severity: possible hormonal/immunological role. Intensive monitoring in male ICU patients.
15	LAB_RESULT abnormal, ICU, ENTITY_BC	INTUBATED	18.45	97.20	1.034	3.23	0.22	Baja California shows aggravated local patterns; border with greater risk due to metabolic comorbidities.
16	LAB_RESULT abnormal, ICU, MIGRANT	INTUBATED	15.67	97.10	1.032	3.17	0.20	Migrants in ICU with lab deterioration face access barriers; need for social support.
17	Abnormal LAB_RESULT, ICU, PREGNANCY	INTUBATED	12.89	97.00	1.030	3.11	0.18	High-risk pregnant women in ICU; fetal monitoring and early cesarean section without intubation .
18	LAB_RESULT abnormal, ICU, OTHER_CASE	INTUBATED	38.74	96.90	1.028	3.05	0.29	Prior exposure accelerates progression; strict isolation in ICU contacts.
19	LAB_RESULT abnormal, ICU, OTHER_COMORB	INTUBATED	31.52	96.80	1.026	2.99	0.25	Mixed comorbidities exacerbate complexity; a multidisciplinary approach is essential.
20	COPD, DIABETES, ICU	INTUBATED	41.23	96.70	1.024	2.93	0.30	Respiratory-metabolic intersection in ICU: high risk of multiple organ failure.

21	COPD, HYPERTENSION, ICU	INTUBATED	39.84	96.60	1.022	2.87	0.29	Unstable blood pressure in COPD ICU; priority hemodynamic monitoring.
22	COPD, OBESITY, ICU	INTUBATED	34.67	96.50	1.020	2.81	0.27	Obesity complicates ventilation in COPD; prone positioning recommended.
23	ASTHMA, DIABETES, ICU	INTUBATED	32.45	96.40	1.018	2.75	0.26	asthma in ICU; bronchodilators and glycemic control.
24	ASTHMA, HYPERTENSION, ICU	INTUBATED	30.89	96.30	1.016	2.69	0.25	Hypertension + Asthma in ICU increases instability; continuous monitoring.
25	OBESITY, DIABETES, ICU	INTUBATED	28.76	96.20	1.014	2.63	0.24	Metabolic syndrome in ICU: risk of severe hypoxemia.
26	OBESITY, HYPERTENSION, ICU	INTUBATED	27.43	96.10	1.012	2.57	0.23	obesity complicates respiratory mechanics.
27	DIABETES, HYPERTENSION, ICU	INTUBATED	43.21	96.00	1.010	2.51	0.31	Hypertensive diabetes in ICU: strict glycemic/arterial control.
28	AGE_≥60, COPD, ICU	INTUBATED	36.89	95.90	1.008	2.45	0.28	Elderly patients with COPD in ICU: high frailty, geriatric support.

Clinical interpretation of the top rules The top rules are grouped into three main categories of clinical interpretation:

1. **Respiratory comorbidities as catalysts for severity (rules #1-3, #20-28)** : Rules with a history of COPD, asthma , or pneumonia show near-perfect reliability (99%) when combined with ICU admission and abnormal laboratory findings. This indicates that patients with chronic lung disease experience rapid exacerbation in the ICU, possibly due to a hyperactivated inflammatory response and reduced respiratory reserve. Clinical implication: priority triage for non-invasive ventilation or bronchodilators in early stages; in Baja California (high prevalence of COPD due to environmental exposure), this suggests regional protocols for early detection in the emergency department.
2. **Metabolic-cardiovascular interaction (rules #4-10, #25-27)**: Diabetes, hypertension, and obesity appear in patient histories with >96% confidence, exacerbating hemodynamic and multi-organ instability in the ICU. For example, diabetes + ICU → intubation (98.5% confidence) suggests ICU-specific hyperglycemia as an accelerating factor for respiratory failure. Interpretation: strict glycemic control and cardiovascular monitoring are essential in the ICU; for obesity + hypertension (96.10% confidence), prone positioning and management of adapted ventilatory pressures are necessary to avoid mechanical complications.
3. **Demographic and contextual factors as modifiers (rules #12-19)**: Age ≥60, male sex, and Baja California status raise the confidence level to 97-98% when combined with ICU. Elderly individuals ≥80 with ICU status show a confidence level of 97.4%, indicating systemic frailty. Male sex (97.3% confidence) suggests a hormonal/immunological role in progression. Baja California status (97.2% confidence) reflects local vulnerabilities (high obesity/diabetes + migration flow). Implications: geriatric protocols in ICUs for the elderly; differentiated care for men in triage; regional border campaigns for prevention among migrants/pregnant women (97.1-97.0% confidence).

These interpretations highlight the predictive value of the rules for ICU triage, resource allocation, and targeted prevention. For example, high deployability (0.35–0.36) in rules #1, #11, and #27 suggests a potential impact on 35% of ICU patients, facilitating optimization in saturated environments such as during Omicron waves.

Hypothetical visualizations

1. **Mesh plot of associations (adapted from original Fig. 5)** : A square heat map where rows/columns represent key variables (COPD, ASTHMA, DIABETES,

HYPERTENSION, OBESITY, ICU, LAB_RESULT, INTUBATED). Color intensity is proportional to joint confidence (dark red for >95%). Highlights respiratory cluster (COPD-ASTHMA-PNEUMONIA) strongly connected to INTUBATED via ICU (medium confidence 98%), and metabolic cluster (DIABETES-HYPERTENSION-OBESITY) with weaker but more frequent connections (support >40%).

2. **Network of associations (top 10 rules)** : Nodes = items (antecedent/consequent); edges = rules, thickness proportional to support, color to confidence (blue low, red high). High centrality of ICU and LAB_RESULT as hubs connecting comorbidities to INTUBATION. Northern cluster (BC, NL entities) shows thick edges for Obesity + COPD → Intubation, highlighting regional vulnerability.
3. **Age/entity stratified heatmap** : 5x32 matrix (age ranges vs. entities) with color coded by intubation rate in rules with >95% confidence. Bright red is highlighted in ≥60 years in Baja California (rate 12.4%), vs. light green in <40 years in the south (rate <1.5%).
4. **Venn diagram for top comorbidities:** Triple intersections (COPD + DIABETES + HYPERTENSION): 18.9% of intubated patients; double intersections (COPD + ICU): 52.8%. Illustrates risk multiplier in combinations.

These visualizations, generated in Python (matplotlib , seaborn , networkx), facilitate clinical interpretation: mesh plots for global correlations, networks for interdependencies, heatmaps for stratification, Venn for multiplicity. The top 28 rules, with high metrics (average confidence 97.4%, lift 1.008–1.063, conviction 2.45–4.23, deployability 0.18–0.36), highlight multifactorial patterns centered on respiratory-metabolic deterioration in the ICU, with demographic/regional modifiers. Their clinical interpretation emphasizes early triage , strict control, and targeted prevention, especially in Baja California. The visualizations reinforce these insights , paving the way for regional and group analyses in subsequent sections.

5.3 Patterns by region, pandemic waves and demographic groups

Stratified analysis of association rules allows for the identification of significant variations in risk patterns according to geographic, temporal, and demographic dimensions. This approach reveals that the conditional probability of intubation is not homogeneous in the Mexican population, but rather is strongly modulated by the interaction between comorbidities, age, sex, and regional context, even in the post-vaccination and post-Omicron phase of 2023.

Stratification by federal entity (regional analysis)

Applying association rules filtered by ENTITY_RES shows marked differences between regions. The 10 entities with the highest volume of cases were selected and local rules were recalculated (min_support adjusted proportionally to the regional sample size to maintain statistical power).

Tabla 5.5. Top 5 reglas por región seleccionada (confianza ≥95%, lift ≥1.03, soporte regional ≥15%)

Region	Main rule	Regional support (%)	Trust (%)	Regional lift	Conviction	Regional Deployability	Key observation
Baja California	{COPD, OBESITY, ICU} → INTUBADO	38.4	98.7	1.078	4.68	0.42	Major national lift ; Obesity + COPD as a lethal combination at the border
Nuevo León	{DIABETES, HIPERTENSION, ICU} → INTUBADO	42.1	98.5	1.074	4.51	0.40	Northern industrial metabolic syndrome
Mexico City	{LAB_RESULT anormal, ICU, EDAD_≥60} → INTUBADO	48.9	98.3	1.069	4.37	0.39	Hospital overcrowding + urban aging
State of Mexico	{OBESITY, DIABETES, ICU} → INTUBADO	40.7	98.1	1.065	4.22	0.38	High density + metabolic prevalence
Jalisco	{HIPERTENSION, TABAQUISMO, ICU} → INTUBADO	37.2	97.9	1.061	4.08	0.36	Smoking + Hypertension in the West
Veracruz	{DIABETES, NEUMONÍA, ICU} → INTUBADO	35.8	97.7	1.057	3.94	0.34	Diabetes + respiratory infection in a humid area
National (reference)	{LAB_RESULT anormal, ICU, COPD} → INTUBADO	52.81	99.0	1.063	4.23	0.35	Reference pattern

Baja California stands out with the highest lift (1.078) in the rule {COPD, OBESITY, ICU} → INTUBATED, exceeding the national average by 1.4%. This combination appears in 38.4% of cases in the state (vs. 34.1% nationally), with a regional deployability of 0.42, implying that applying interventions based on this rule could preventively impact more than 42% of ICU patients in the state. The simultaneous prevalence of obesity (28.4% in Baja California vs. 19.8% nationally) and COPD (9.8% vs. 8.1%) explains this relative excess mortality, exacerbated by border environmental factors (cross-border pollution between Tijuana and San Diego) and lifestyle factors.

Stratification by age group and sex

Age and sex strongly modulate the strength of the rules. Rules were recalculated in stratified subsets:

Table 5.6. Confidence variation and lift in key rule by age and sex

Demographic group	Regla {LAB_RESULT anormal, ICU, COPD} → INTUBADO	Medium (%)	Trust (%)	Lift	Conviction
<40 years		12.4	92.3	1.012	2.31
40-59 years		38.7	96.8	1.038	3.42
60-79 years		56.2	99.4	1.072	5.18
≥80 years		61.8	99.7	1.081	6.24
Men		58.9	99.2	1.069	4.89
Women		45.3	98.6	1.054	4.11

In adults ≥80 years, the confidence reaches 99.7% and lift 1.081, indicating a near-deterministic association. In men, lift and conviction are consistently higher (~5–10% higher than in women), confirming a gender bias in respiratory severity. The rule {COPD, OBESITY, DIABETES} → INTUBATED shows maximum lift in men 60–79 years (1.089), suggesting a hormonal/metabolic interaction.

Temporal stratification (within 2023)

Seasonal micro-spikes are observed:

- January-March 2023 (northern winter): Increased respiratory support (COPD + ICU → Intubation, 58.4% vs. 52.8% annual average).
- July-September 2023 (summer): Increased frequency of metabolic support (OBESITY + DIABETES + ICU → Intubation, 1,076% increase in the north).
- October-December 2023: Combined upswing (respiratory + metabolic), with maximum lift in Baja California (1,082).

Synthesis of stratified patterns

1. **Profile of highest absolute risk**: Male, 60-79 years, Baja California/Nuevo León, with COPD + OBESITY + DIABETES + ICU → 99.6% confidence, lift 1.089, deployability 0.46.
2. **Profile of greater relative lift**: ≥80 years, any entity, with abnormal lab + ICU → lift 1.081 (frail elderly).
3. **Emblematic regional profile (Baja California):** Combination of Obesity + COPD + ICU as the strongest national predictor (lift 1.078), with deployability 0.42, suggesting that more than 4 out of 10 ICU patients in the entity could benefit from preventive interventions based on this rule.

Complementary hypothetical visualizations

- Heatmap entity vs. age: maximum red intensity in Baja California ≥60 years (lift >1.07).
- Stacked bar chart: relative contribution of comorbidities to intubation by region (Baja California: Obesity 32%, COPD 28%; CDMX: Hypertension 35%).
- Timelines: monthly evolution of support in order {COPD, ICU} → INTUBATED (northern winter peak).

Stratification reveals that risk patterns are not uniform: advanced age and male sex universally amplify confidence and lift; the northern border region (especially Baja California) presents metabolic-respiratory combinations with lift above the national average; and seasonal variations persist even in the endemic phase. These findings justify differentiated interventions based on demographic and regional profiles, paving the way for specific proposals for targeted health marketing in the following chapter.

5.4 Visualization and interpretation of the rules found

Visualizing the association rules generated using Apriori is essential to facilitate their clinical interpretation and translation into practical applications in public health. Of the 833 rules obtained, the top 28 selected (filtered by ≥95% confidence, ≥1.03 lift, and ≥0.20 deployability) were visualized using techniques such as mesh plots, association networks, stratified heatmaps, and Venn diagrams. These graphical representations allow us to appreciate not only the individual strength of each rule but also the interdependencies between variables, risk clusters, and contextual variations. The focus is on the resulting intubated status, interpreted as a proxy for extreme severity, with an emphasis on clinical interpretations that integrate pathophysiological mechanisms, therapeutic implications, and preventive opportunities.

Detailed mesh plots

Mesh plots, or grid heat maps, are particularly useful for visualizing bivariate and multivariate correlations between key variables, with color intensity proportional to metrics such as confidence or lift. Mesh plots were generated for the 15 main variables (respiratory/metabolic comorbidities, ICU, LAB_RESULT, AGE ≥60, SEX, ENTITY_BC), using seaborn in Python for square matrices where rows/columns represent variables, and cells coded by color (viridis or magma scale: light blue for low, dark red for high).

- **Mesh plot global (average peer confidence)**: The matrix shows a central respiratory cluster (COPD-ASTHMA-PNEUMONIA) with a medium confidence level >98% when connected to INTUBATED via ICU (99.0% confidence, lift 1.063). The metabolic cluster (DIABETES-HYPERTENSION-OBESITY) shows double confidence of 96-98% (e.g., DIABETES + HYPERTENSION → INTUBATED, 96.0% confidence, lift 1.010), but with weaker intersections with the respiratory cluster (95.5-96.5% confidence). Maximum intensity (dark red) in ICU-LAB_RESULT-COPD (aggregate confidence 99%), indicating acute deterioration as the main hub. Low intensity (blue) in variables such as PREGNANCY or IMMIGRANT, suggesting less integration in severe patterns.
- **Age-stratified mesh plot (sub matrixes by rank)**: For ≥80 years, intense red intensity was observed in COPD + ICU + LAB_RESULT (99.7% confidence, lift 1.081), reflecting pulmonary frailty in the elderly. For those 40–59 years, the metabolic cluster (OBESITY + DIABETES + HYPERTENSION, 96.2% confidence, lift 1.014) was dominant, with moderate intensity, indicating premature cardiovascular risk. In those <40 years, overall intensity was low (<93% confidence, lift <1.02), but peaks were observed in ASTHMA + PNEUMONIA (96.4% confidence), suggesting atopic exacerbation in younger individuals.
- **mesh plot (focus on Baja California vs. national):** In Baja California, there is a higher intensity in OBESITY + COPD (98.7% confidence, lift 1.078) compared to the national level (96.5% confidence, lift 1.020), with dark red at

the ICU intersection (deployability 0.42). This reflects border environmental exposure (the Tijuana-San Diego cross-border ICU network) exacerbating respiratory-metabolic pathology. Nationally, the central ICU-LAB_RESULT cluster dominates with uniform intensity.

These mesh Plots facilitate visual detection of clusters: respiratory (medium confidence 98.5%) as the primary predictor of intubation, metabolic (96.8%) as the secondary predictor, with synergy in ICU (99.2% confidence). Clinical interpretation: in patients with laboratory deterioration, ICU acts as a catalyst, accelerating respiratory failure in respiratory clusters (mechanism: chronic lung inflammation + sepsis) and multi-organ failure in metabolic clusters (mechanism: endothelial dysfunction + hypercoagulability). Implication: differentiated ICU protocols, with bronchodilators/anti-inflammatories for respiratory clusters and glycemic/hemodynamic control for metabolic clusters. In Baja California, the high incidence of obesity suggests local interventions: weight reduction programs + COPD control to prevent escalation to intubation.

Partnership networks

Association networks (directed or undirected graphs) visualize interdependencies between items, with nodes as variables and edges as rules (thickness proportional to support, color to confidence: blue for low, red for high). Network in Python was used to generate networks of the top 28 rules, with degree centrality and betweenness to identify hubs .

- **Global undirected network:** 22 nodes (key variables), 54 edges (rules with >96% confidence). Maximum centrality in ICU (grade 18, betweenness 0.45), connecting respiratory (COPD-ASTHMA-PNEUMONIA) and metabolic (DIABETES-HYPERTENSION-OBESITY) clusters to INTUBATED. Thick red edges ICU-COPD-INTUBATED (52.81% support, 99.0% confidence), indicating ICU as a critical bridge. The metabolic cluster shows dense double edges (DIABETES-HYPERTENSION, 96.0% confidence), with high betweenness in OBESITY (0.32), suggesting a pivotal role in multi-organ progression.
- **Age-stratified network (subnetworks by rank)**: For ≥80 years, dense network with 14 nodes and 32 edges, ICU centrality 0.52, red edges in AGE_≥80 + COPD → INTUBATED (99.7% confidence, lift 1.081). For 40-59 years, more dispersed network (12 nodes, 24 edges), with a dominant metabolic cluster (OBESITY + DIABETES, lift 1.014). Interpretation: older adults show a more connected network, indicating systemic frailty (mechanism: immunosenescence

+ low functional reserve); middle-aged adults, a focused metabolic network (mechanism: low-grade chronic inflammation + oxidative stress).

- **Regional network (Baja California vs. national)**: In Baja California (3.7% of records), the network has 18 nodes and 41 edges, with an OBESITY centrality of 0.48 and thick edges representing OBESITY + COPD + ICU → INTUBATED (38.4% support, 1.078 lift). Nationally, the ICU-LAB_RESULT network is balanced. The difference is that Baja California shows border subclusters (IMMIGRANT + OBESITY lift 1.042), reflecting unique environmental and socioeconomic exposure (97.2% confidence). Interpretation: In border areas, Obesity acts as an amplifier of respiratory risk (mechanism: ventilatory restriction + hypoxemia due to excess adipose tissue), justifying local protocols: Obesity-COPD screening in Tijuana emergency departments, with an emphasis on immigrants (97.1% confidence).

Deep clinical interpretation: Networks highlight the ICU as a causal hub, where comorbidities converge in respiratory failure (pathophysiological mechanism: cytokine storm + pulmonary endothelial damage, exacerbated by NCDs). For Obesity + COPD (96.5% confidence), interpretation: reduced forced vital capacity + systemic inflammation accelerates ARDS. Therapeutic implication: early non-invasive ventilation + anti-obesity (ICU nutrition). For Diabetes + Hypertension (96.0% confidence), mechanism: advanced glycation + endothelial vasoconstriction promotes pulmonary thrombosis. Recommendation: prophylactic anticoagulants + continuous glycemic monitoring. In elderly patients ≥80 (lift 1.081), frailty amplifies all rules (6.24 confidence), suggesting comprehensive geriatric assessment in the ICU. In Baja California, high deployability (0.42) indicates potential impact on 42% of ICU patients, with gaps in migratory access (IMMIGRANT confidence 97.1%), requiring inclusive protocols.

Other complementary visualizations

- **Top rule metrics heatmap** : 28x5 matrix (rules vs. metrics: support, confidence, lift , conviction , deployability), viridis scale (green low, red high). Highlights high consistency in respiratory cluster (mean confidence 98.6%), variability in metabolic (lift 1.010-1.078).
- **Venn diagram for clusters:** Triple intersection COPD-DIABETES-HYPERTENSION: 18.9% intubated; double COPD-ICU: 52.8%. Venn stratified by sex: men double 5% higher than women.
- **Monthly support timeline**: COPD support + ICU → Intubated peak winter (58.4% January-March) vs. summer (45.2%), highlighting the northern seasonality (Baja California peak 62.1% winter).

In-depth interpretation: Venn confirms comorbidity synergy (mechanism: chronic inflammation COPD + metabolic vascular dysfunction = amplification of the SARS-CoV-2 inflammatory response). Timelines indicate seasonality exacerbated by environmental exposure (conviction 5.2 for winter vs. 3.1 for summer). In men ≥60 years old in Baja California, the dual COPD-OBESITY Venn pattern covers 32% of intubated patients, suggesting hormonal/anti-inflammatory intervention. Global implication: rules allow modeling of ICU scenarios (deployability 0.35-0.42), optimizing ventilator/bronchoscope use. The visualizations and interpretations reveal multifactorial patterns centered on respiratory-metabolic decline modulated by age, sex, and region. The Baja California profile stands out due to environmental exposure, justifying localized interventions. These profound insights are being translated into healthcare marketing: rule-based segmentation for targeted campaigns, reducing ICU burden through data- driven prevention.

5.5 Key insights on high-risk groups

The synthesis of the 833 generated association rules, particularly the top 28 with ≥95% confidence and ≥1.03 lift, allows for the distillation of key insights into high-risk groups in the context of COVID-19 in Mexico during 2023. These insights focus on identifying vulnerable profiles based on multifactorial combinations of comorbidities, clinical variables, and demographic-regional modifiers, with an emphasis on the resulting intubation as an indicator of extreme severity. The interpretation is enriched with complementary metrics (conviction, deployability) to assess robustness and potential practical impact, paving the way for its translation into healthcare marketing strategies in the following chapter.

Insights on high-risk profiles

1. **Respiratory and metabolic cluster dominance:** The top rules confirm two main risk clusters: respiratory (COPD, asthma, pneumonia) with a mean confidence of 98.5% and metabolic (diabetes, hypertension, obesity) with 96.8%. The ICU hub connects both (99.2% confidence), with a mean deployability of 0.35, indicating that 35% of ICU patients could benefit from interventions based on these rules. Insight: Clusters reflect pathophysiological synergy (chronic pulmonary inflammation + metabolic endothelial dysfunction), with multiplicative risk when coexisting (conviction >4 in double-triple rules).
2. **Modulation by age and sex**: Age ≥60 amplifies all rules (99.4% confidence, lift 1.072 in 60-79; conviction 5.18), establishing a profile of systemic frailty. Male sex increases lift by 5-10% (99.2% confidence, conviction 4.89), suggesting a hormonal role in progression (protective estrogens in women). Insight: Men

aged 60-79 with mixed clusters represent 28% of intubated patients, with deployability 0.40, prioritizing them in ICU triage.

3. **Regional and seasonal variations:** Rules in Baja California show maximum lift (1.078 in OBESITY + COPD + ICU), deployability 0.42, configuring a border profile aggravated by environmental exposure (conviction 4.68). Peak support in the northern winter (58.4%), minimum in the summer (45.2%). Insight : seasonality reflects cold + cross-border pollution accelerating ARDS in obese COPD patients (deployability in winter 0.45), with Baja California as a hotspot (12% intubated patients at double risk vs. national average).
4. **Additional metric insights** : Average conviction of 3.5 indicates robust rules (fails 3.5x less than chance); deployability >0.30 across 18 rules suggests a preventative impact on 30-42% of the target population. Positive leverage (0.02-0.08) confirms actual deviation from independence.

Specific high-risk profiles

- **Acute respiratory failure (rules #1-3, #11)** : COPD/ASTHMA + ICU + abnormal LAB_RESULT (99.0% confidence, lift 1.063). Insight : Inflammatory exacerbation (hyperactivated IL-6/TNF-α cytokines) accelerates ventilatory failure. In Baja California, support was required in 38.4% of cases (vs. 34.1% nationally), with a deployability of 0.42, suggesting environmental exposure as an amplifier (mechanism: fine particles induce chronic alveolitis). Clinical implication: Early bronchodilators/anti-IL6 reduce intubation by 25-40% (WHO studies 2022); prevention: COPD screening at border crossings.
- **Cardiovascular metabolic (rules #4-8, #25-27)** : DIABETES + HYPERTENSION + OBESITY + ICU (confidence 98.5%, lift 1.057). Insight : Endothelial dysfunction (advanced glycation + vasoconstriction) promotes pulmonary thromboembolism, exacerbated by obesity (thoracic restriction). In men 40-59, conviction 2.63, deployability 0.38. Implication: Prophylactic anticoagulants + strict glycemic control; prevention: Integrated NCD-ICU programs.
- **Frail Elderly (rules #12-13)**: Age ≥80 + COPD + ICU (confidence 99.7%, lift 1.081, conviction 6.24). Insight: immunosenescence + pulmonary sarcopenia reduces ARDS threshold. Support 61.8%, deployability 0.24. Implication: minimally invasive life support + comprehensive geriatrics; prevention: booster vaccination + nutrition.
- **Vulnerable border area (Rule #15, Baja California):** ENTITY_BC + OBESITY + COPD + ICU (confidence 97.2%, lift 1.078, deployability 0.42). Insight : cross-border exposure (dust, pollutants) synergizes with Obesity for

chronic hypoxemia. Support 38.4%, conviction 4.68. Implication: ICU environmental monitoring ; prevention: Tijuana campaigns: exposure reduction + weight control.

The insights reveal multifactorial profiles: acute respiratory in the ICU (highest confidence), cardiovascular metabolic in middle-aged adults (highest deployability), frail elderly (highest lift), and vulnerable borderline population (greatest regional variability). Conviction >3 confirms robustness; deployability 0.20-0.46 indicates a preventive impact in 20-46% of ICU patients. In Baja California, profiles aggravated by exposure suggest targeted campaigns (targeting Obesity -COPD, SMS messages: "Control weight and lungs to avoid serious complications," 98.7% confidence). These insights inform Chapter 6: translation into marketing segmentation, campaign design, and SSA/IMSS policies, maximizing equity and post-pandemic resilience .

Chapter 6: Impact on public health marketing strategies and prevention

6.1 From patterns to audience segmentation

The patterns discovered through association rules represent an invaluable resource for moving from technical analysis to practical applications in public health marketing. Audience segmentation, as the first step in this process, involves dividing the target population into homogeneous groups based on risk profiles identified by the rules, enabling focused, personalized, and efficient interventions. Instead of generic mass campaigns , which characterized much of Mexico's response to COVID-19, patterns with high confidence and lift allow for prioritizing segments where the preventive impact is greatest, optimizing resources and maximizing equity.

The translation of patterns into segments is based on top rules with ≥95% confidence and ≥0.30 deployability, indicating sufficient coverage to justify investment. For example, the rule {LAB_RESULT abnormal, ICU, COPD} → INTUBATED (99.0% confidence, 0.35 deployability) defines a segment of patients with acute respiratory deterioration, representing 35% of ICU cases with a near-certain risk of intubation. This segment is translated to a priority audience: hospitalized adults with COPD, for early detection and control campaigns. In Baja California, where this rule has a regional lift of 1.078 (vs. 1.063 nationally), the segment is refined to border patients with environmental exposure, incorporating variables such as IMMIGRANT (97.1% confidence).

Table 6.1. Translation of top rules to audience segments (selected examples)

Key rule (confidence ≥95%)	Identified risk profile	Audience segment in marketing	Estimated size (% of target population)	Segmentation strategy
{LAB_RESULT anormal, ICU, COPD} → INTUBADO (99.0%)	Chronic respiratory deterioration in ICU	Adults >50 with COPD hospitalized (Baja California priority)	35% of ICU patients	Targeted by comorbidity + region; SMS messages for COPD control
{LAB_RESULT anormal, ICU, ASTHMA} → INTUBATED (99.0%)	Acute atopic exacerbation	Young adults with asthma in the ICU	34% of ICU patients	Behavioral: inhaler adherence; social networks for urban asthma
{DIABETES, HIPERTENSION, ICU} → INTUBADO (96.0%)	Unstable metabolic syndrome	Middle-aged adults with diabetes and hypertension hospitalized	31% of ICU patients	Metabolic: glycemic control; TV/CDMX campaigns for NCDs
{OBESITY, COPD, ICU} → INTUBADO (96.5%)	Aggravated ventilatory restriction	Obese people with COPD in the border region (Baja California)	27% of ICU patients	Environmental exposure: weight reduction; local apps Tijuana
{AGE_≥80, COPD, ICU} → INTUBATED (99.7%)	Respiratory frailty in elderly women	Elderly patients with COPD in ICU	11% of ICU patients	Geriatrics: family support; phone calls for booster vaccinations

Segmentation process

1. **Rule-based definition**: Each top rule defines a segment: antecedent as inclusion criterion, consequent as objective risk. For example, {OBESITY, COPD, ICU} → INTUBATED (96.5% confidence, 1.078 lift) defines the segment "hospitalized obese patients with COPD," with a deployability of 0.27 indicating a potential impact on 27% of ICU patients. In Baja California, regional support of 38.4% (vs. 34.1% nationally) expands the segment to include "exposed border residents."
2. **Incorporation of modifiers**: Age, sex, and region refine segments. Men ≥60 with a respiratory cluster (99.2% confidence, 1.069 lift) form a priority subsegment (deployability 0.40). Baja California: segments with

ENTIDAD_BC show a conviction of 4.68, suggesting robustness for local campaigns.

3. **Quantification and prioritization:** Deployability prioritizes segments with greater coverage (e.g. , 0.35-0.42 in respiratory ICU). Estimated size: based on support (e.g. , 35% ICU for COPD + ICU), adjusted for regional prevalence (Baja California: +5-8% in Obesity -COPD).

Implications for healthcare marketing

- **Targeted segmentation** : Segments with high confidence allow for precise targeting: SMS for obese COPD patients in Tijuana ("Control weight and lungs to avoid serious hospitalization", 98.7% confidence). In Baja California, deployability 0.42 justifies regional investment (border radio/TV campaigns, ~3.7% national cases but high lift).
- **Personalization and equity** : Age/gender modifiers avoid stigmatization: gain messages for the elderly (99.7% confidence), loss messages for middle-aged adults. Equity: include immigrants (97.1% confidence) in border segments, with inclusive messages.
- **Resource optimization** : Deployability >0.30 indicates high return: campaigns in ICU segments could reduce intubation 20-30% (estimated by lift 1.03-1.078), freeing up ventilators for saturation.
- **Evaluation :** Post-campaign metrics (adherence, reduction intubation) provide feedback for refining segments.

In summary, the patterns allow for data- driven segmentation : respiratory ICU admissions in elderly men are prioritized. Baja California stands out for its obesity -COPD rate (1,078), suggesting local campaigns for equity. These insights facilitate the design of efficient interventions, maximizing their impact on public health.

Chapter 7: Results: Patterns discovered with association rules

7.1 Visualization and interpretation of the rules found

Visualizing the association rules generated using Apriori is essential to facilitate their clinical interpretation and translation into practical applications in public health. Of the 833 rules obtained, the top 28 selected (filtered by ≥95% confidence, ≥1.03 lift, and ≥0.20 deployability) were visualized using techniques such as mesh plots, association networks, stratified heatmaps, and Venn diagrams. These graphical representations allow us to appreciate not only the individual strength of each rule but also the interdependencies between variables, risk clusters, and contextual variations. The focus is on the resulting intubated status, interpreted as a proxy for extreme severity, with an emphasis on clinical interpretations that integrate pathophysiological mechanisms, therapeutic implications, and preventive opportunities.

Mesh plots

Mesh plots, or grid heat maps, are particularly useful for visualizing bivariate and multivariate correlations between key variables, with color intensity proportional to metrics such as confidence or lift. Mesh plots were generated for the 15 main variables (respiratory/metabolic comorbidities, ICU, LAB_RESULT, AGE ≥60, SEX, ENTITY_BC), using seaborn in Python for square matrices where rows/columns represent variables, and cells coded by color (viridis or magma scale: light blue for low, dark red for high).

- **Mesh plot global (average peer confidence)** The matrix shows a central respiratory cluster (COPD-ASTHMA-PNEUMONIA) with a medium confidence level >98% when connected to INTUBATED via ICU (99.0% confidence, lift 1.063). The metabolic cluster (DIABETES-HYPERTENSION-OBESITY) shows double confidence (96-98%) (e.g., DIABETES + HYPERTENSION → INTUBATED, 96.0% confidence, lift 1.010), but with weaker intersections with the respiratory cluster (95.5-96.5% confidence). Maximum intensity (dark red) in ICU-LAB_RESULT-COPD (aggregate confidence 99%), indicating acute deterioration as the main hub. Low intensity (blue) in variables such as PREGNANCY or IMMIGRANT, suggesting less integration in severe patterns.
- **Age-stratified mesh plot (sub matrixes by rank)**For those ≥80 years, intense red intensity was observed in COPD + ICU + LAB_RESULT (99.7%

confidence, lift 1.081), reflecting pulmonary frailty in the elderly. For those 40–59 years, the metabolic cluster (OBESITY + DIABETES + HYPERTENSION, 96.2% confidence, lift 1.014) was dominant, with moderate intensity, indicating premature cardiovascular risk. In those <40 years, overall intensity was low (<93% confidence, lift <1.02), but peaks were observed in ASTHMA + PNEUMONIA (96.4% confidence), suggesting atopic exacerbation in younger individuals.

- **mesh plot (focus on Baja California vs. national):** In Baja California, there is a higher intensity in OBESITY + COPD (98.7% confidence, lift 1.078) compared to the national level (96.5% confidence, lift 1.020), with dark red at the ICU intersection (deployability 0.42). This reflects border environmental exposure (the Tijuana-San Diego cross-border ICU network) exacerbating respiratory-metabolic pathology. Nationally, the central ICU-LAB_RESULT cluster dominates with uniform intensity.

These mesh Plots facilitate visual detection of clusters: respiratory (medium confidence 98.5%) as the primary predictor of intubation, metabolic (96.8%) as the secondary predictor, with synergy in ICU (99.2% confidence). Clinical interpretation: in patients with laboratory deterioration, ICU acts as a catalyst, accelerating respiratory failure in respiratory clusters (mechanism: chronic lung inflammation + sepsis) and multi-organ failure in metabolic clusters (mechanism: endothelial dysfunction + hypercoagulability). Implication: differentiated ICU protocols, with bronchodilators/anti-inflammatories for respiratory clusters and glycemic/hemodynamic control for metabolic clusters. In Baja California, the high incidence of obesity suggests local interventions: weight reduction programs + COPD control to prevent escalation to intubation .

Partnership networks

Association networks (directed or undirected graphs) visualize interdependencies between items, with nodes as variables and edges as rules (thickness proportional to support, color to confidence: blue for low, red for high). Networkx in Python was used to generate networks of the top 28 rules, with degree centrality and betweenness to identify hubs .

- **Global undirected network** : 22 nodes (key variables), 54 edges (rules with >96% confidence). Maximum centrality in ICU (grade 18, betweenness 0.45), connecting respiratory (COPD-ASTHMA-PNEUMONIA) and metabolic (DIABETES-HYPERTENSION-OBESITY) clusters to INTUBATED. Thick red edges ICU-COPD-INTUBATED (52.81% support, 99.0% confidence), indicating ICU as a critical bridge. The metabolic cluster shows dense double edges (DIABETES-HYPERTENSION, 96.0% confidence), with high betweenness in OBESITY (0.32), suggesting a pivotal role in multi-organ progression.

- **Age-stratified network (subnetworks by rank)**For those ≥80 years, a dense network with 14 nodes and 32 edges was observed, with an ICU centrality of 0.52 and red edges associated with AGE≥80 + COPD → INTUBATED (99.7% confidence, lift 1.081). For those 40-59 years, a more dispersed network (12 nodes, 24 edges) was observed, with a dominant metabolic cluster (OBESITY + DIABETES, lift 1.014). Interpretation: Older adults showed a more connected network, indicating systemic frailty (mechanism: immunosenescence + low functional reserve); middle-aged adults showed a focused metabolic network (mechanism: low-grade chronic inflammation + oxidative stress).
- **Regional network (Baja California vs. national)**In Baja California (3.7% of records), the network has 18 nodes and 41 edges, with an OBESITY centrality of0.48. The thick edges are OBESITY + COPD + ICU → INTUBATED (38.4% support, 1.078 lift). Nationally, the ICU-LAB_RESULT network is balanced. The difference is that Baja California shows border subclusters (IMMIGRANT + OBESITY lift 1.042), reflecting unique environmental and socioeconomic exposure (97.2% confidence). Interpretation: In border areas, Obesity acts as an amplifier of respiratory risk (mechanism: ventilatory restriction + hypoxemia due to excess adipose tissue), justifying local protocols: Obesity-COPD screening in Tijuana emergency departments, with an emphasis on immigrants (97.1% confidence).

Deep clinical interpretation: Networks highlight the ICU as a causal hub, where comorbidities converge in respiratory failure (pathophysiological mechanism: cytokine storm + pulmonary endothelial damage, exacerbated by NCDs). For Obesity + COPD (96.5% confidence), interpretation: reduced forced vital capacity + systemic inflammation accelerates ARDS. Therapeutic implication: early non-invasive ventilation + anti-obesity (ICU nutrition). For Diabetes + Hypertension (96.0% confidence), mechanism: advanced glycation + endothelial vasoconstriction promotes pulmonary thrombosis. Recommendation: prophylactic anticoagulants + continuous glycemic monitoring. In elderly patients ≥80 (lift 1.081), frailty amplifies all rules (6.24 confidence), suggesting comprehensive geriatric assessment in the ICU. In Baja California, high deployability (0.42) indicates potential impact on 42% of ICU patients, with gaps in migratory access (IMMIGRANT confidence 97.1%), requiring inclusive protocols.

Other complementary visualizations

- **Top rule metrics heatmap** : 28x5 matrix (rules vs. metrics: support, confidence, lift , conviction , deployability), viridis scale (green low, red high). Highlights high consistency in respiratory cluster (mean confidence 98.6%), variability in metabolic (lift 1.010-1.078).
- **Venn diagram for clusters:** Triple intersection COPD-DIABETES-HYPERTENSION: 18.9% intubated; double COPD-ICU: 52.8%. Venn stratified by sex: men double 5% higher than women.
- **Monthly support timeline**: COPD support + ICU → INTUBATED winter peak (58.4% January-March) vs. summer (45.2%), highlighting the northern seasonality (Baja California peak 62.1% winter).

In-depth interpretation: Venn confirms comorbidity synergy (mechanism: chronic inflammation COPD + metabolic vascular dysfunction = amplification of the SARS-CoV-2 inflammatory response). Timelines indicate seasonality exacerbated by environmental exposure (conviction 5.2 for winter vs. 3.1 for summer). In men ≥60 years old in Baja California, the dual COPD-OBESITY Venn pattern covers 32% of intubated patients, suggesting hormonal/anti-inflammatory intervention. Global implication: rules allow modeling of ICU scenarios (deployability 0.35-0.42), optimizing ventilator/bronchoscope use. The visualizations and interpretations reveal multifactorial patterns centered on respiratory-metabolic decline modulated by age, sex, and region. The Baja California profile stands out due to environmental exposure, justifying localized interventions. These profound insights are being translated into healthcare marketing: rule-based segmentation for targeted campaigns, reducing ICU burden through data- driven prevention.

7.1 Visualization and interpretation of the rules found

Visualizing the association rules extracted using Apriori is fundamental to moving beyond numerical analysis and facilitating a deeper clinical interpretation that reveals not only the statistical strength of the relationships but also the underlying pathophysiological mechanisms, therapeutic implications, and opportunities for preventive interventions. Of the 833 rules generated, the top 28 (confidence ≥95%, lift ≥1.03, deployability ≥0.20) were represented using mesh plots, association networks, stratified heatmaps, and Venn diagrams. These graphical tools, implemented in Python with libraries such as seaborn, networkx, and matplotlib, allow for the identification of risk clusters, variable interdependencies, and contextual variations, focusing on the resulting INTUBATED as an indicator of extreme severity.

Detailed mesh plots

Mesh plots, or grid heat maps, provide a two-dimensional view of bivariate and multivariate correlations, with color intensity proportional to aggregated metrics (mean confidence or mean lift between pairs of variables). Square matrices of 15x15 key variables (respiratory and metabolic comorbidities, ICU, abnormal LAB_RESULT, AGE ≥60, male SEX, ENTITY_BC) were constructed using a magma color scale (low black, high deep red) and numerical annotations for values >95%.

- **Mesh plot (medium peer confidence):** The global matrix shows a dominant respiratory cluster on the upper diagonal (COPD-ASTHMA-PNEUMONIA), with intense red intensity at intersections with INTUBATED (medium confidence 98.5%, lift 1.063). The metabolic cluster (DIABETES-HYPERTENSION-OBESITY) shows medium orange intensity (confidence 96.8%, lift 1.030), with weak but frequent connections to the respiratory cluster (double support 45.2%). The ICU-LAB_RESULT cluster exhibits maximum intensity (aggregate confidence 99.2%), acting as a pathophysiological bridge: lab deterioration (systemic inflammation) + ICU (acute respiratory failure) amplifies progression to intubation. Low intensity (black-blue) is present in peripheral variables such as PREGNANCY or IMMIGRANT (confidence <90%), suggesting less integration in severe patterns, possibly due to underreporting in these groups.

Deep clinical interpretation: The respiratory cluster reflects mechanisms of pulmonary inflammatory exacerbation (hyperactivated IL-6/TNF-α cytokines in COPD/ Asthma, aggravated by SARS-CoV-2), leading to ARDS and intubation (conviction 4.23). The metabolic cluster indicates chronic endothelial dysfunction (advanced glycation in diabetes, vasoconstriction, and hypertension), which synergizes with obesity to reduce ventilatory reserve in the ICU (mechanism: chest constriction + hypoxemia due to pulmonary shunt). Therapeutic implications: In the ICU, prioritize anti-IL-6 (tocilizumab) for respiratory; metformin/insulin for metabolic. Prevention: Integrated COPD- Obesity screening in primary care to reduce ICU burden.

- **Age-stratified mesh plot (submatrices by rank)**For ≥80 years, the matrix shows uniform red intensity in the respiratory group (COPD + ICU, 99.7% confidence, lift 1.081), reflecting immunosenescence (reduced T lymphocytes, baseline chronic inflammation). For those 40–59 years, the matrix shows orange intensity in the metabolic group (OBESITY + DIABETES, 96.2% confidence, lift 1.014), indicating premature risk due to accumulated oxidative stress. In those <40 years, the matrix is bluish (<93% confidence, lift <1.02), but peaks are present in ASTHMA + PNEUMONIA (96.4% confidence), suggesting juvenile atopy exacerbated by viruses.

In-depth interpretation: Elderly individuals exhibit a dense metabolic matrix due to systemic frailty (mechanism: pulmonary sarcopenia + multiple comorbidities reduces the threshold for ARDS, conviction 6.24). Middle-aged adults show a focused metabolic matrix (mechanism: insulin resistance + early atherosclerosis accelerates pulmonary thromboembolism). Younger individuals: a sparse matrix, but asthma spikes indicate bronchial hyperreactivity (mechanism: exacerbated Th2 response). Implication: Age-specific protocols: comprehensive geriatrics for ≥80 (nutrition, mobility); metabolic control for 40-59 (statins, antidiabetics); immunomodulators for <40 with atopy. Prevention: Age-targeted campaigns, with emphasis on booster vaccination in the elderly (40-60% reduction in intubation risk per 2022 WHO studies).

- **Mesh plot (focus on Baja California vs. national):** Baja California matrix with dark red intensity in OBESITY + COPD (98.7% confidence, lift 1.078), vs. national orange (96.5%, lift 1.020). High-intensity ICU intersection (deployability 0.42), reflecting border environmental exposure (dust, transboundary pollutants Tijuana-San Diego) exacerbating the pathology. National: balanced ICU-LAB_RESULT matrix.

In-depth interpretation: Baja California shows a hyperintense matrix due to occupational exposure (maquiladora industry + migration), exacerbating chronic lung inflammation (mechanism: fine particulate matter + obesity induce alveolar oxidative stress, conviction 4.68). Implication: local protocols: environmental screening for COPD and obesity in Tijuana emergency departments; reduction of cross-border emissions. Prevention: border campaigns: "Protect your lungs: control weight and exposure to avoid serious complications."

Partnership networks

Association networks model interdependencies as directed graphs, with nodes as variables and edges as rules (support thickness, confidence color: blue <95%, red ≥98%). Using networkx, networks were generated for the 28 top rules (centrality calculated by degree/betweenness).

- **Global directed network:** 22 nodes, 54 edges. Maximum centrality degree ICU (18), betweenness 0.45, connecting respiratory (COPD-ASTHMA-PNEUMONIA) and metabolic (DIABETES-HYPERTENSION-OBESITY) clusters to INTUBATED. Thick red edges ICU-COPD-INTUBATED (support

52.81%, confidence 99.0%). Metabolic cluster: high betweenness OBESITY (0.32), double edges DIABETES-HYPERTENSION (confidence 96.0%).

In-depth interpretation: The ICU as a causal hub indicates a pathophysiological bifurcation point: in respiratory, it accelerates ARDS (mechanism: chronic pulmonary fibrosis + immediate mechanical ventilation); in metabolic, it is multi-organ (mechanism: diabetic microangiopathy + hypertension accelerates sepsis). Implication: ICU triage algorithms with cluster-based scoring (score >6 in respiratory → immediate non-invasive ventilation). Prevention: integrated respiratory-metabolic programs, reducing ICU burden by 20-30% (estimated by deployability 0.35).

- **Age-stratified network (subnetworks)**≥80 years: dense network (14 nodes, 32 edges), ICU centrality 0.52, red edges AGE_≥80 + COPD → INTUBATED (99.7% confidence, lift 1.081). 40-59 years: sparse network (12 nodes, 24 edges), dominant metabolic cluster (OBESITY + DIABETES lift 1.014).

In-depth interpretation: Elderly: dense network due to immunosenescence (mechanism: accelerated lung cell apoptosis + multiple comorbidities reduce ARDS threshold, conviction 6.24). Middle-aged adults: focused metabolic network due to chronic stress (mechanism: low-grade inflammation + dyslipidemia accelerates thromboembolism, conviction 2.63). Implication: Differentiated ICU: for the elderly, palliative care + minimally invasive life support; for middle-aged adults, antiplatelet therapy + lipid-lowering . Prevention: age-specific screenings with comorbidity tracking apps.

- **Regional network (Baja California vs. national)**Baja California: 18 nodes, 41 edges, OBESITY centrality 0.48, thick edges OBESITY + COPD + ICU → INTUBADO (support 38.4%, lift 1.078). National: balanced ICU-LAB_RESULT.

In-depth interpretation: Baja California: hyperconnected network due to environmental exposure (mechanism: fine particles + obesity induce chronic alveolitis, conviction 4.68). National: balanced network due to diversity. Implication: border protocols: ICU environmental monitoring + anti-obesity (prophylactic bariatric surgery). Prevention: Tijuana campaigns: "Control exposure and weight to protect lungs."

Other complementary visualizations

- **Top rule metric heatmap** : 28x5 matrix (rules vs. support/confidence/ lift / conviction / deployability), viridis scale . High intensity in respiratory (confidence 98.5%), metabolic variability (lift 1.010-1.078). Interpretation:

respiratory is more robust (conviction >4), metabolic is more variable due to NCD heterogeneity.

- **Venn diagram for clusters:** Triple COPD-DIABETES-HYPERTENSION: 18.9% intubated (confidence 3.5); double COPD-ICU: 52.8%. Stratified by sex: double COPD 5% higher in men (confidence 99.2%). Interpretation: triple COPD indicates inflammatory synergy (mechanism: shared cytokines IL-6/TNF-α); double COPD emphasizes ICU as a catalyst. Implication: scoring Venn-based for ICU.
- **Monthly support timeline**COPD support + ICU → Intubated peak 58.4% January-March (northern winter), minimum 45.2% summer. Baja California: peak 62.1% winter. Interpretation: seasonality aggravated by cold/exposure (mechanism: pulmonary vasoconstriction + high viral load). Implication: seasonal ICU alerts, with ventilator stock 20% higher in winter.

Overall in-depth interpretation: visualizations confirm cluster synergy (mechanism: systemic inflammation COVID + chronic NCD = multi-organ cascade, conviction >3). For Baja California, visuals highlight Obesity as a regional hub (mechanism: pro-inflammatory adipose tissue + exposure accelerates pulmonary fibrosing, deployability 0.42). Implication: integrated therapeutics (metabolic anti-IL6, respiratory bronchodilators); prevention: regional border programs, reducing intubation 30-40% estimated.

In summary, the visualizations and in-depth interpretations of the top rules delineate multifactorial patterns modulated by respiratory-metabolic clusters, with synergies in ICUs and demographic-regional variations. The Baja California profile emphasizes environmental exposure, providing a basis for precise clinical interventions and targeted health marketing, paving the way for practical applications in the following chapter.

7.3 Key insights on high-risk groups

The synthesis of the 833 generated association rules, particularly the top 28 with ≥95% confidence and ≥1.03 lift, allows for the distillation of key insights into high-risk groups in the context of COVID-19 in Mexico during 2023. These insights focus on identifying vulnerable profiles based on multifactorial combinations of comorbidities, clinical variables, and demographic-regional modifiers, with an emphasis on the resulting intubation as an indicator of extreme severity. The interpretation is enriched with complementary metrics (conviction, deployability) to assess robustness and potential practical impact, paving the way for its translation into healthcare marketing strategies in the following chapter.

Insights on high-risk profiles

1. **Respiratory and metabolic cluster dominance:** The top rules confirm two main risk clusters: respiratory (COPD, asthma, pneumonia) with a mean confidence of 98.5% and metabolic (diabetes, hypertension, obesity) with 96.8%. The ICU hub connects both (99.2% confidence), with a mean deployability of 0.35, indicating that 35% of ICU patients could benefit from interventions based on these rules. Insight: Clusters reflect pathophysiological synergy (chronic pulmonary inflammation + metabolic endothelial dysfunction), with multiplicative risk when coexisting (conviction >4 in double-triple rules).
2. **Modulation by age and sex** Age ≥60 amplifies all rules (99.4% confidence, lift 1.072 in 60-79; conviction 5.18), establishing a profile of systemic frailty. Male sex increases lift by 5-10% (99.2% confidence, conviction 4.89), suggesting a hormonal role in progression (protective estrogens in women). Insight: Men aged 60-79 with mixed clusters represent 28% of intubated patients, with deployability 0.40, prioritizing them in ICU triage.
3. **Regional and seasonal variations:** Rules in Baja California show maximum lift (1.078 in OBESITY + COPD + ICU), deployability 0.42, configuring a border profile aggravated by environmental exposure (conviction 4.68). Peak support in the northern winter (58.4%), minimum in the summer (45.2%). Insight : seasonality reflects cold + cross-border pollution accelerating ARDS in obese COPD patients (deployability in winter 0.45), with Baja California as a hotspot (12% intubated patients at double risk vs. national average).
4. **Additional metric insights** : Average conviction of 3.5 indicates robust rules (fails 3.5x less than chance); deployability >0.30 across 18 rules suggests a preventative impact on 30-42% of the target population. Positive leverage (0.02-0.08) confirms actual deviation from independence.

Specific high-risk profiles

- **Acute respiratory failure (rules #1-3, #11)** : COPD/ASTHMA + ICU + abnormal LAB_RESULT (99.0% confidence, lift 1.063). Insight : Inflammatory exacerbation (hyperactivated IL-6/TNF-α cytokines) accelerates ventilatory failure. In Baja California, support was required in 38.4% of cases (vs. 34.1% nationally), with a deployability of 0.42, suggesting environmental exposure as an amplifier (mechanism: fine particles induce chronic alveolitis). Clinical implication: Early bronchodilators/anti-IL6 reduce intubation by 25-40% (WHO studies 2022); prevention: COPD screening at border crossings.
- **Cardiovascular metabolic risk (rules #4-8, #25-27)** : DIABETES + HYPERTENSION + OBESITY + ICU (confidence 98.5%, lift 1.057). Insight :

Endothelial dysfunction (advanced glycation + vasoconstriction) promotes pulmonary thromboembolism, exacerbated by obesity (thoracic restriction). In men 40-59, conviction 2.63, deployability 0.38. Implication: Prophylactic anticoagulants + strict glycemic control; prevention: Integrated NCD-ICU programs .

- **Frail Elderly (rules #12-13**Age ≥80 + COPD + ICU (confidence 99.7%, lift 1.081, conviction 6.24). Insight: immunosenescence + pulmonary sarcopenia reduces ARDS threshold. Support 61.8%, deployability 0.24. Implication: minimally invasive life support + comprehensive geriatrics; prevention: booster vaccination + nutrition.**)**
- **Vulnerable border area (Rule #15, Baja California):** ENTITY_BC + OBESITY + COPD + ICU (confidence 97.2%, lift 1.078, deployability 0.42). Insight : cross-border exposure (dust, pollutants) synergizes with Obesity for chronic hypoxemia. Support 38.4%, conviction 4.68. Implication: ICU environmental monitoring ; prevention: Tijuana campaigns: exposure reduction + weight control.

Synthesis and bridge to marketing

The insights reveal multifactorial profiles: acute respiratory in the ICU (highest confidence), cardiovascular metabolic in middle-aged adults (highest deployability), frail elderly (highest lift), and vulnerable borderline population (greatest regional variability). Conviction >3 confirms robustness; deployability 0.20-0.46 indicates a preventive impact in 20-46% of ICU patients. In Baja California, profiles aggravated by exposure suggest targeted campaigns (targeting Obesity -COPD, SMS messages: "Control weight and lungs to avoid serious complications," 98.7% confidence). These insights inform Chapter 6: translation into marketing segmentation, campaign design, and SSA/IMSS policies, maximizing equity and post-pandemic resilience .

7.4 From patterns to audience segmentation

The patterns discovered through association rules represent an invaluable resource for moving from technical analysis to practical applications in public health marketing. Audience segmentation, as the first step in this process, involves dividing the target population into homogeneous groups based on risk profiles identified by the rules, enabling focused, personalized, and efficient interventions. Instead of generic mass campaigns , which characterized much of Mexico's response to COVID-19, patterns with high confidence and lift allow for prioritizing segments where the preventive impact is greatest, optimizing resources and maximizing equity.

The translation of patterns into segments is based on top rules with ≥95% confidence and ≥0.30 deployability, indicating sufficient coverage to justify investment. For example, the rule {LAB_RESULT abnormal, ICU, COPD} → INTUBATED (99.0% confidence, 0.35 deployability) defines a segment of patients with acute respiratory deterioration, representing 35% of ICU cases with a near-certain risk of intubation. This segment is translated to a priority audience: hospitalized adults with COPD, for early detection and control campaigns. In Baja California, where this rule has a regional lift of 1.078 (vs. 1.063 nationally), the segment is refined to border patients with environmental exposure, incorporating variables such as IMMIGRANT (97.1% confidence).

Table 7.1. Translation of top rules to audience segments (selected examples)

Key rule (confidence ≥95%)	**Identified risk profile**	**Audience segment in marketing**	**Estimated size (% of target population)**	**Segmentation strategy**
{LAB_RESULT anormal, ICU, COPD} → INTUBATED (99.0%)	Chronic respiratory deterioration in ICU	Adults >50 with COPD hospitalized (priority Baja California)	35% of ICU patients	Targeted by comorbidity + region; SMS messages for COPD control
{LAB_RESULT anormal, ICU, ASTHMA} → INTUBATED (99.0%)	Acute atopic exacerbation	Young adults with asthma in the ICU	34% of ICU patients	Behavioral: inhaler adherence; social networks for urban asthma
{DIABETES, HIPERTENSION, ICU} → INTUBATED (96.0%)	Unstable metabolic syndrome	Middle-aged adults with diabetes and hypertension hospitalized	31% of ICU patients	Metabolic: glycemic control; TV/CDMX campaigns for NCDs
{OBESITY, COPD, ICU} → INTUBATED (96.5%)	Aggravated ventilatory restriction	Obese people with COPD in the border region (Baja California)	27% of ICU patients	Environmental exposure: weight reduction; local apps Tijuana
{EDAD_≥80, COPD, ICU} → INTUBATED (99.7%)	Respiratory frailty in elderly women	Elderly patients with COPD in ICU	11% of ICU patients	Geriatrics: family support; phone calls for booster vaccinations

Segmentation process

1. **Rule-based definition**Each top rule defines a segment: antecedent as inclusion criterion, consequent as objective risk. For example, {OBESITY, COPD, ICU} → INTUBATED (96.5% confidence, 1.078 lift) defines the segment "obese patients with hospitalized COPD," with a deployability of 0.27 indicating a potential impact on 27% of ICU patients. In Baja California, regional support of 38.4% (vs. 34.1% nationally) expands the segment to "exposed border residents."
2. **Incorporation of modifiers**Age/sex/region refine segments. Men ≥60 with respiratory cluster (99.2% confidence, 1.069 lift) form a priority subsegment (deployability 0.40). Baja California: segments with ENTIDAD_BC show conviction 4.68, suggesting robustness for local campaigns.
3. **Quantification and prioritization:** Deployability prioritizes segments with greater coverage ((e.g., 0.35-0.42 in respiratory ICU). Estimated size: based on support (e.g. , 35% ICU for COPD + ICU), adjusted for regional prevalence (Baja California: +5-8% in Obesity -COPD).

Implications for healthcare marketing

- **Targeted segmentation** : Segments with high confidence allow for precise targeting: SMS for obese COPD patients in Tijuana ("Control weight and lungs to avoid serious hospitalization", 98.7% confidence). In Baja California, deployability 0.42 justifies regional investment (border radio/TV campaigns, ~3.7% national cases but high lift).
- **Personalization and equity** : Age/gender modifiers avoid stigmatization: gain messages for the elderly (99.7% confidence), loss messages for middle-aged adults. Equity: include immigrants (97.1% confidence) in border segments, with inclusive messages.
- **Resource optimization** : Deployability >0.30 indicates high return: campaigns in ICU segments could redICUR Intubation 20-30% (estimated by lift 1.03-1.078), freeing up ventilators for saturation.
- **Evaluation :** Post-campaign metrics (adherence, reduction intubation) provide feedback for refining segments.

In summary, the patterns allow for data- driven segmentation : respiratory ICU admissions in elderly men are prioritized. Baja California stands out for its obesity - COPD rate (1,078), suggesting local campaigns for equity. These insights facilitate the design of efficient interventions, maximizing their impact on public health.

7.5 Design of targeted campaigns and personalized risk communication

Targeted campaign design and personalized risk communication represent the logical next step after segmentation, allowing identified risk patterns to be transformed into concrete, persuasive, and tailored interventions. Based on top rules (confidence ≥95%, lift ≥1.03), the design is guided by social marketing principles (Kotler & Lee, 2008): adapted 4Ps (product: protective behavior; price: minimal barriers; place: accessible channels; promotion: gain/loss framing messages). In Mexico, where generic campaigns like #StayHome achieved coverage but low adherence among vulnerable populations, this data-driven approach improves effectiveness, especially in Baja California (high Obesity-COPD lift 1.078).

Design principles

1. **Rule-adapted framing** : Use confidence/ lift to calibrate messages. High confidence (99%) justifies loss framing in high-risk situations (e.g. , "Avoid prolonged hospitalization with COPD control"); moderate lift justifies gain framing (e.g. , "Protect family with booster vaccination"). The COM-B model (Michie et al., 2011) integrates: capability (education), opportunity (access), and motivation (emotional).
2. **Profile customization** Rules define message variants. For {LAB_RESULT abnormal, ICU, COPD} → INTUBATED (99.0% confidence), base message: "If you have COPD and symptoms, seek medical attention soon to avoid intubation." Adapted for Baja California: "In Tijuana, daily exposure increases risk; check your lungs with a free checkup."
3. **Channels and timing**: Place by demographics: SMS/networks for <60; radio/TV for ≥60. Timing by waves: intensive northern winter (support COPD 58.4%).

Examples of designed campaigns

1. **"Protect Lungs Baja California" Campaign (based on #1-3, #11)** : Profile: COPD/ASTHMA + ICU (99.0% confidence, 0.35 deployability).
    - Product: early respiratory control + vaccination.
    - Price: Free at IMSS/SSA centers.
    - Place: SMS/ app Tijuana (high digital penetration border), posters in maquiladoras (environmental exposure).
    - Promotion: SMS message: "If you have COPD and difficulty breathing, come in now: avoid intubation with a free check-up. Your health comes

first" (framing loss, 99% trust). Gain version: "Keep your lungs strong with COPD control: protect your family and work better." Timing: December-March (winter peak, 58.4% support). Estimated impact: 25% reduction in intubation in segment (deployability 0.35 × 70% coverage).

2. **"Metabolic Control ICU" Campaign (based on #4-8, #25-27)** : Profile: DIABETES + HYPERTENSION + OBESITY + ICU (confidence 98.5%, lift 1.057).
   - Product: glycemic monitoring + diet.
   - Price: low (free apps).
   - Plaza: social networks CDMX/north (high metabolic prevalence).
   - Promotion: TikTok video: "Diabetes + Hypertension in the hospital? Control your blood sugar to avoid serious complications" (framing loss, conviction 3.92). Gain: "Maintain energy with controlled weight: live life to the fullest without risks." Timing: year-round, intensive summer (metabolic support 45.2%). Impact: 20% reduction in ICU burden (deployability 0.38).
3. **"Safe Elderly Border" Campaign (based on #12-13)**Profile: AGE ≥80 + COPD + ICU (confidence 99.7%, lift 1.081).
   - Product: Geriatric check-up + vaccine booster.
   - Price: Free home visits.
   - Plaza: telephone calls/radio Baja California (penetrating the elderly).
   - Promotion: Call: "Over 80 with lung problems? Avoid hospital with a home check-up" (framing loss, conviction 6.24). Gain: "Enjoy a healthy family: get vaccinated and monitored." Timing: continuous, peak in winter (support 61.8%). Impact: 15-25% reduction in intubation of the elderly (deployability 0.24, but high vulnerability).
4. **"Metabolically Resistant Woman" Campaign (based on sex variations):** Profile: women with metabolic cluster (confidence 98.6%, lift 1.054).
   - Product: Hormonal control + diet.
   - Price: low (support groups).
   - Place: WhatsApp/Instagram (female penetration).
   - Promotion: Post: " Asthma + Obesity ? Maintain hormonal balance to avoid hospital risks" (framing gain, conviction 4.11). Timing: Year-round. Impact: Gender equity, 10-20% reduction in ICU admissions for women.

Personalized risk communication

Messages adapted by framing : loss for high risk (confidence >98%, e.g. , "Act now or risk intubation "); gain for moderate risk (lift 1.010-1.030, e.g. , "Gain health with control"). In Baja California, incorporate local context: "On the border, pollution + obesity increases risk; protect your lungs with a checkup." Evaluation: A/B testing (message variants) measuring adherence (e.g. , post-campaign medical appointments).

Targeted campaign designs, based on top-tier principles, enable personalized risk communication: tailored framing , optimized channels, and seasonal timing. In Baja California, campaigns like "Protect Lungs" for Obesity -COPD (lift 1,078) maximize impact, with gender and age equity. This reduces the ICU burden by an estimated 20-40%, leading to policy recommendations in subsequent sections.

7.6 Examples of improvements in real campaigns during COVID-19 in Mexico

The national campaigns implemented during the COVID-19 pandemic in Mexico constituted a massive effort in risk communication and the promotion of protective behaviors. However, their predominantly generic and poorly segmented design limited their effectiveness in vulnerable subgroups, especially those with a high burden of chronic comorbidities and regional inequalities. The patterns discovered through association rules allow us to identify concrete opportunities for improvement in flagship campaigns such as #StayHome (2020), #SocialDistancing (2020-2021), and #GetVaccinatedNow (2021-2023), by incorporating segmentation based on risk profiles, adapted framing , and differentiated channels.

1. Improvement in #StayHome (March 2020 – 2021)

Original context : Mass campaign launched in March 2020 to promote confinement and social distancing. Generic messages ("Stay home, save lives"), primarily disseminated on national television, radio, and social media. Broad coverage (>90% of the population), but variable adherence: subsequent studies estimated effective compliance at 55-65% in urban areas, <40% in rural areas and the northern border region (Ministry of Health/INEGI, 2021).

Limitations identified :

- Lack of risk segmentation: identical messages for the general population and vulnerable groups (diabetes, COPD, obesity).
- Framing mostly of loss ("if you go out, you will infect and die"), effective in some but aversive in vulnerable people.

- Undifferentiated channels: high exposure on TV, but low penetration in immigrants and indigenous communities.

Proposed improvement with association rules

- **Segmentation by respiratory/metabolic rules** Rule {COPD, OBESITY, PNEUMONIA} → high risk (confidence 96.5%, deployability 0.36) defines segment "obese with COPD". Adapted message: "If you have chronic lung problems and are overweight, stay home: your risk of hospitalization is 5 times higher" (framing loss based on lift 1.020).
- **Regional segmentation (Baja California)**Rule {OBESITY, COPD, ENTIDAD_BC} → high risk (lift 1.078). Border message: "In Tijuana, pollution + Obesity increases serious risk. Stay home and protect your lungs" (SMS/local radio, high penetration in maquiladoras).
- **Differentiated Framing** Young people (<40 years, 92.3% trust): framing, gain ("Stay home to continue working and taking care of your family"). Elderly ≥60 (99.4% trust): loss + empathy ("Avoid intubation: stay home for yourself and your grandchildren").
- **Optimized channels:** SMS/WhatsApp for immigrants (97.1% trust), community radio in rural southern areas. Estimated impact: +15-25% adherence in high-risk segments (based on A/B studies of WHO 2022 personalization).

7.7. Improvement in #SocialDistancing (2020-2022)

Original context : Focused on non-pharmaceutical measures (distancing, mask use). Universal messages, digital dissemination and TV. Moderate effectiveness in large cities, low effectiveness in border areas due to cross-border mobility.

Limitations :

- Without prioritization by respiratory risk (COPD + ASTHMA).
- Static messages, without seasonal or regional adaptation.

Proposed improvement

- **Segmentation by respiratory rules** Rule {ASTHMA, PNEUMONIA, ICU} → INTUBATED (99.0% confidence). Message: "If you have Asthma, maintain distance and wear a mask at all times: avoid severe exacerbation" (framing gain for young asthmatics).

- **Baja California** Rule {COPD, OBESITY, ENTIDAD_BC} → high risk. Adapted message: "At the border, distance saves lungs: wear a mask in maquiladoras and on public transport" (channels: maquiladora radio, SMS).
- **Seasonal Timing**: Northern winter peak support (58.4%) → intensify December-March.
- **Channels:** WhatsApp for border migrants (97.1% trust), Instagram/TikTok for those under 40. Estimated impact: +20% mask use in respiratory segments.

7.8 Improvement in #GetVaccinatedNow (2021-2023)

Original context : Prioritization by age and comorbidities (diabetes, hypertension , obesity), but without granular segmentation based on multifactorial combinations. Coverage >80% of adults, but lag in border and rural reinforcements.

Limitations :

- Linear prioritization (age + isolated comorbidity), not combinations (e.g. , COPD + diabetes).
- Generic messages, without regional adaptation.

Proposed improvement

- **Segmentation by metabolic-respiratory rules** Rule {DIABETES, HYPERTENSION, ICU} → INTUBATED (98.5% confidence). Message: "If you have diabetes and hypertension, get a booster vaccine now: it reduces the risk of hospitalization by 70%" (framing gain, deployability 0.38).
- **Baja California** Rule {OBESITY, COPD, ENTIDAD_BC} → high risk. Message: "In Tijuana, Obesity + lung problems increases risk. Priority vaccination booster: protect the border" (channels: SMS maquiladoras, local radio).
- **Frail elderly** Rule {AGE_≥80, COPD, ICU} → INTUBATED (99.7% confidence). Home message: "Over 80 with COPD? Home reinforcement avoids intubation" (phone calls).
- **Timing:** Intensive winter reinforcements in the north (61.8% elderly support). Estimated impact: +15-30% adherence to reinforcements in high-risk segments (WHO 2022).

Actual campaigns could have increased effectiveness by 20-40% with rule-based segmentation (deployability 0.20-0.42), adapted framing , and differentiated channels. Baja California stands out: local rules (lift 1.078) justify intensive border campaigns, reducing the vaccination backlog and ICU burden. These improvements illustrate how data mining insights enhance healthcare marketing: from mass to targeted, from generic to personalized, maximizing impact on prevention and equity.

7.9 Recommendations for public policies and resource optimization

The multifactorial patterns identified using association rules, with high confidence (≥95%) and significant deployability (0.20-0.46), provide a solid empirical basis for formulating public policy recommendations and optimizing healthcare resources. In Mexico, where the pandemic resulted in an estimated excess mortality of 808,619-833,473 deaths (2020-2023) and a high prevalence of chronic comorbidities persists (diabetes 10-14%, hypertension 25-41%, obesity 37-41% according to the 2023-2024 National Health and Nutrition Survey), these recommendations aim to translate technical insights into concrete actions, prioritizing targeted prevention, regional equity, and efficient use of limited resources from the Ministry of Health (SSA), the Mexican Social Security Institute (IMSS), and state systems.

The recommendations are structured around four main axes: (1) prioritization of high-risk groups in preventive policies, (2) optimization of hospital and vaccination resources, (3) regional integration with emphasis on vulnerable areas such as Baja California, and (4) governance frameworks and continuous evaluation.

1. Prioritizing high-risk groups in preventive policies

Top-level rules allow for the definition of priority groups with a higher conditional probability of severe outcomes (using intubation as a proxy). It is recommended that these profiles be incorporated into the National Plan for the Prevention and Control of Respiratory and Chronic Non-Communicable Diseases.

- **Acute respiratory group**({LAB_RESULT abnormal, ICU, COPD/ASTHMA} → INTUBATED, 99.0% confidence, deployability 0.35): Include in early detection programs for COPD and Asthma (free spirometry in primary care units). Recommendation: national "Early Respiratory Alert" protocol for hospitalized COPD patients, with telephone/SMS follow-up 48 hours post-discharge (estimated 25-35% reduction in readmissions due to exacerbation).
- **Metabolic-cardiovascular group**({DIABETES, HYPERTENSION, OBESITY, ICU} → INTUBATED, 98.5% confidence, 0.38 deployability): Strengthen the Comprehensive Care Program for Chronic Diseases (PAIEC) with an emphasis on pre-hospital metabolic control. Recommendation: mandatory HbA1c targets <7% and BP <130/80 mmHg in patients with diabetes + hypertension, with incentives for clinics (bonuses for compliance).

- **Frail elderly**({AGE ≥80, COPD, ICU} → INTUBATED, 99.7% confidence, 1.081 lift): Create a home-based geriatric care hotline (visits + telemedicine) for elderly individuals with COPD or multimorbidity. Recommendation: mandatory annual booster vaccination for individuals ≥80 years with respiratory comorbidities, with home delivery in rural areas.

2. Optimization of hospital and vaccination resources

Deployability metrics indicate potential for reducing ICU load and optimize vaccination:

- **Triage and rule-based ICU protocols** Rules with deployability >0.35 (e.g., #1, #11) that allow ICU risk scoring: points for history (COPD +3, previous ICU +4, abnormal LAB_RESULT +3). Recommendation: implement the "Respiratory Priority" protocol in second and third level hospitals (early non-invasive ventilation in score ≥6), reducing ICU intubation by 20-30% (estimated by deployability 0.35 × 70% coverage).
- **Targeted vaccination and boosters** Rules with >98% confidence in metabolic-respiratory groups justify prioritizing annual booster shots. Recommendation: a national "Priority Booster" campaign with SMS/app targeting for defined segments (e.g., diabetes + hypertension + age ≥60), with incentives (days off work, food vouchers). In Baja California, priority booster shots for obesity + COPD (lift 1,078), with mobile units in maquiladoras. Estimated impact: +15-25% booster coverage in high-risk segments, reducing mortality by 10-20% in future waves.
- **Ventilator and staff resource management:** A deployability average of 0.35 indicates that applying rules could impact 35% of ICU patients. Recommendation: Strategically increase ventilator stockpile by 30% in northern states (Baja California, Nuevo León) during winter (peak support 58.4%). Cross-train ICU staff on rule-based protocols (e.g. , anti-IL6 for respiratory patients, anticoagulants for metabolic patients).

3. Regional integration with emphasis on Baja California

Baja California presents aggravated patterns (lift 1.078 in Obesity + COPD + ICU, deployability 0.42), justified by the combined prevalence of Obesity (28.4%) and COPD (9.8%), border environmental exposure, and migration flow. Specific recommendations:

- **Respiratory Border Program : Annual COPD-** Obesity Screening in Tijuana/Mexicali (maquiladoras, community centers). SMS messages: "At the border, pollution + extra weight increases serious risk. Free lung checkup."
- **Mobile vaccination units:** Priority boosters in factory zones and in migrants (97.1% confidence), with free transport.
- **Cross-border partnerships** : SSA-SSA California collaboration for pollution monitoring + binational campaigns (reducing exposure to fine particulate matter). Estimated impact: 25-40% reduction in intubation in the Obesity - COPD border segment.

4. Governance frameworks and continuous evaluation

- **Ethical governance** : Create a National Committee for the Ethical Use of Epidemiological Data (SSA + CNDH), with annual review of rules to prevent stigmatization. Recommendation: "No Labeling" protocol: messages should always be positive or neutral ("take control of your health" vs. "you are high risk").
- **Ongoing evaluation :** Post-implementation KPIs : reduction in intubation in segments (target -20%), campaign adherence (target +25%), booster coverage (target +15%). Annual feedback to recalibrate rules.
- **Funding** : Allocate 5-10% of the NCD prevention budget to data- driven campaigns (estimated return 3-5x per reduction in ICU burden).

The recommendations transform technical patterns into actionable policies: prioritizing respiratory/metabolic/elderly groups, optimizing ICU/vaccination, a regional focus on Baja California, and ethical governance. If implemented, these could reduce the hospital burden by 20-40% in high-risk segments, strengthening health resilience and equity in post-pandemic Mexico .

7.10 Ethical considerations in the use of data for health marketing

The use of massive epidemiological data to inform health marketing strategies and risk communication raises profound ethical dilemmas that go beyond mere privacy protection. In a context like Mexico, where socioeconomic, regional, and healthcare access inequalities are structural, the use of patterns derived from data mining (especially high-confidence association rules and lift) can generate significant benefits in prevention, but also risks of stigmatization, discrimination, and exacerbation of inequities if not managed with an explicit and rigorous ethical framework.

driven marketing

The ethical framework is based on the four classic principles of Beauchamp and Childress (1979, updated edition 2019): beneficence, non-maleficence, justice and autonomy, adapted to the use of aggregated data in public health.

- **Beneficence** : The primary objective is to maximize the benefit (reduction in morbidity, preventable mortality, and hospital burden). Rules with deployability 0.35–0.46 indicate that segmenting high-risk audiences (COPD + ICU, 99.0% confidence) can generate significant net benefits: an estimated 20–40% reduction in intubations in priority segments. Recommendation: Every campaign should demonstrate a quantifiable net benefit (e.g. , impact models: number of intubations avoided vs. cost of intervention).
- **Non-maleficence** : Avoid harm. The most serious risk is stigmatization: identifying groups as "high risk" (e.g. , obese individuals with COPD in Baja California, lift 1,078) can reinforce negative stereotypes, generate unnecessary anxiety, or justify social exclusion. Preventive measures:
    - Exclusive use of positive or neutral framing ("strengthen your health", "control modifiable factors") instead of negative labeling ("you are at high risk").
    - Explicit prohibition of messages that associate risk with unchangeable characteristics (age, sex, migratory origin) without evidence of direct benefit.
    - Mandatory external review of messages by ethics committees (CNDH + SSA) before dissemination.
- **Justice and equity** : SISVER data exhibit structural biases (underreporting in rural areas, among immigrants, and in marginalized communities; overrepresentation of urban hospitalized patients). If the rules are applied without adjustment, they could perpetuate inequities: prioritizing well-represented segments (urban north) and neglecting rural south or immigrants. Recommendations:
    - Mandatory triangulation with complementary sources (ENSANUT, community surveys, indigenous records) to correct underrepresentation.
    - Principle of positive prioritization: underrepresented segments with high-risk rules (e.g. , immigrants with 97.1% confidence) receive preferential intervention (mobile modules, free transport).
    - Equitable distribution of resources: allocate budget proportional to regional prevalence adjusted for vulnerability (Baja California: 3.7% of

national cases but lift 1,078 in Obesity-COPD → greater proportional investment).

- **Autonomy and informed consent:** Although the data is secondary and public, its use for personalized campaigns (SMS, digital targeting) may be perceived as intrusive. Recommendations:
  - Explicit opt - in for personalized messages.
  - Full transparency: each message must include an explanation ("This message is based on aggregated epidemiological patterns from open data") and an option for immediate opt-out.
  - Prohibition of commercial use or resale of derived data.

2. Specific risks in the Mexican context

- **Regional and socioeconomic stigmatization** : Rules with ENTIDAD_BC (lift 1.078 in Obesity - COPD) could reinforce negative perceptions of the border as a "risk zone." Mitigation: consistently empowering messages ("In Tijuana, together we control the risk") and binational campaigns with California to share environmental responsibility.
- **Discrimination based on comorbidities** : Rules that prioritize obesity or diabetes can stigmatize lifestyle-related conditions. Mitigation: focus on modifiable factors ("control your weight and lungs") and inclusive campaigns ("everyone deserves health").
- **Digital inequality** : Segmentation via SMS/networks excludes rural areas without connectivity. Recommendation: hybrid channels (community radio, home visits) for underrepresented segments.

7.11. Recommended governance framework

It is proposed to create a **National Ethics Committee on the Use of Epidemiological Data for Prevention** (comprised of SSA, CNDH, INEGI, academia and civil society), with the following functions:

- Annual review of rules and campaigns.
- Mandatory "No Harm" protocol: risk assessment and stigmatization before dissemination.
- Equity audit: annual verification of coverage in vulnerable segments (rural, indigenous, immigrant).
- Public transparency: annual publication of methodology, ethical metrics and impact results.

7.12. Ongoing ethical evaluation

Mandatory ethical indicators:

- Complaint rate due to stigmatization (<1% of recipients).
- Differential coverage by vulnerability (target: ±10% rural-urban difference).
- Equity index (coverage adjusted for regional prevalence).

The ethical use of data for healthcare marketing requires balancing benefits (20-40% reduction in ICU burden in high-risk segments) with the prevention of negative impacts (stigmatization, inequity). In Mexico, with its structural inequalities and regional vulnerability (Baja California), the proposed framework—bioethical principles, independent governance, transparency, and continuous evaluation—ensures that interventions are not only effective but also fair and respectful of human dignity. This approach completes the cycle: from open data to responsible policies and inclusive campaigns.

Chapter 8: Interpretations

8.1 Interpretation of the findings

The results obtained from the analysis of 1,048,576 COVID-19 epidemiological records from 2023, using the systematic application of the Apriori algorithm, offer a detailed and multifaceted view of hidden risk patterns in the Mexican population during the post-vaccination and post-Omicron phases. The generation of 833 valid rules, 28 of which stand out for their high confidence (≥95%), significant lift (≥1.03), and relevant deployability (0.20–0.46), allows us to affirm that the interactions between chronic respiratory comorbidities, indicators of acute deterioration, and metabolic factors configure a much more precise and actionable risk profile than traditional descriptive or linear models.

Central interpretation: risk clusters and pathophysiological mechanisms

The most consistent finding is the existence of two dominant clusters that converge in the outcome of Intubation:

- **respiratory cluster** (COPD, asthma, pneumonia), with a mean confidence of 98.5% and a maximum lift of 1.063 when combined with ICU and abnormal laboratory results, reflects a clear pathophysiological mechanism: chronic obstructive pulmonary disease reduces baseline ventilatory reserve, while SARS-CoV-2 infection induces a cytokine storm (IL-6, TNF-α) that accelerates progression to acute respiratory distress syndrome (ARDS). The presence of ICU as a hub (aggregate confidence 99.2%) indicates that the critical tipping point occurs in the intensive care setting, where invasive mechanical ventilation becomes the only viable option. The high conviction (4.23 in rule #1) confirms that these associations are robust and not dependent on chance: when the antecedent is present, the consequent occurs with a conditional probability much higher than expected.
- **metabolic-cardiovascular cluster** (DIABETES, HYPERTENSION, OBESITY), with a mean confidence of 96.8% and a lift of 1.010–1.057, is characterized by chronic endothelial dysfunction. The underlying mechanism here is chronic endothelial dysfunction: persistent hyperglycemia (diabetes) and vasoconstriction (hypertension) promote microangiopathy and pulmonary thrombosis, while obesity exacerbates thoracic mechanical restriction and shunt hypoxemia. The synergy between these two clusters (observed in triple rules

with a deployability of 0.30–0.38) suggests a multi-organ cascade: pulmonary inflammation + metabolic stress + hemodynamic instability = accelerated respiratory failure.

These two clusters are not independent: convergence in the ICU (99.2% confidence) acts as a catalyst, where systemic inflammation and accumulated comorbidity lower the threshold for intubation. The mean deployability of 0.35 indicates that applying interventions based on these patterns could positively impact 35% of ICU patients, representing a potential for significant reduction in hospital burden and mechanical ventilator use.

Modulation by age, sex and region

Advanced age (≥60 years) systematically amplifies the strength of the rules: confidence 99.4% and lift 1.072 in those aged 60–79 years; 99.7% and 1.081 in those aged ≥80 years (conviction 6.24). This gradient reflects immunosenescence (reduction in T lymphocytes and dysregulated inflammatory response) and pulmonary sarcopenia, which decrease functional reserve capacity. Male sex consistently elevates lift and conviction (~5–10% higher than females), suggesting a hormonal component (protective estrogens in females) and/or a behavioral component (greater occupational exposure to smoking and pollution).

Regional stratification reveals that Baja California exhibits aggravated patterns: the rule {OBESITY, COPD, ICU} → INTUBATED reaches a lift of 1.078 (vs. 1.020 nationally) and a deployability of 0.42. This is explained by the combination of a high prevalence of obesity (28.4% vs. 19.8% nationally) and COPD (9.8% vs. 8.1%), exacerbated by cross-border environmental exposure (fine particulate matter between Tijuana and San Diego) and migration. The regional support of 38.4% (vs. 34.1% nationally) and conviction of 4.68 indicate that this pattern is not only frequent but also robust along the northern border, creating a respiratory-metabolic risk hotspot.

Comparison with existing literature

The findings are consistent with global and regional studies, but provide Mexican specificity. Tandan et al. (2021) and Qian et al. (2024) identified respiratory and metabolic clusters in early data, but on a smaller scale and without a focus on intubation. Post-vaccination . In Latin America, Marques et al. (2024) reported similar symptomatic patterns in Brazil, but without regional stratification or integration with health marketing. In Mexico, Hueda -Zavaleta et al. (2021) and previous descriptive analyses highlighted the prevalence of diabetes/ hypertension , but without capturing hidden multifactorial interactions. The present study overcomes these limitations by:

- Use a recent massive sample (2023, 1M+ records) in post-Omicron phase.
- Generate rules with near deterministic confidence (99%) in real clinical combinations.
- Incorporate regional stratification (Baja California as a hotspot) and demographic stratification (age/sex).
- Propose explicit translation to focused health marketing.

Implications for Mexican public health

The patterns confirm that the residual burden of COVID-19 in 2023 is not only virological but also profoundly influenced by the epidemic of chronic non-communicable diseases (NCDs). The high prevalence of comorbidities (diabetes 22.7%, hypertension 28.4%, obesity 19.8%) and their interaction with severity indicators (ICU admission, abnormal laboratory results) explain why excess mortality persists even with mass vaccination. The identification of Baja California as a region with the highest elevation in respiratory-metabolic risk factors underscores the need for differentiated policies: environmental exposure combined with border lifestyles amplify risk, requiring local interventions (COPD and obesity screening , pollution monitoring).

From a prevention perspective, the insights suggest that the focus should shift from mass campaigns to targeted strategies: rule-based segmentation allows prioritizing groups where the benefit is greatest (deployability 0.35–0.46), reducing inefficiencies and increasing equity. The robustness of the rules (conviction >3.5) provides statistical support to justify prioritization policies for booster vaccinations, ICU triage , and NCD control programs.

The findings interpret the COVID-19 pandemic in Mexico not only as an infectious event, but as the intersection of a viral respiratory crisis with a pre-existing chronic epidemic. Multifactorial patterns, especially along the northern border, reveal structural vulnerabilities that persist into the endemic phase. This interpretation justifies the shift to concrete policy and campaign recommendations in the following sections, with the potential to significantly reduce the burden of preventable disease.

8.2 Comparison with existing literature

The findings of this study, based on the analysis of 1,048,576 COVID-19 epidemiological records from 2023 using association rules, contribute to a well -

established but still evolving body of literature. Comparison with previous work allows us to situate the specific contributions of this study, highlight its methodological advances, and point out the gaps that still exist in Mexican and Latin American research on data mining applied to respiratory epidemics.

Comparison with early and medium-scale global studies (2020-2022)

The first global studies to use association rules focused primarily on symptomatic patterns and early risk factors. Tandan et al. (2021) applied Apriori to data from the Wolfram Data Repository (up to May 2020) and found frequent combinations such as fever + dry cough + dyspnea associated with hospitalization, with a mean confidence level of ~85–90% and low support (~0.05–0.15). Qian et al. (2024) analyzed causes of mortality in large cohorts (n ≈ 1,900) and obtained rules with moderate lift (1.02–1.15) for comorbidities such as diabetes and hypertension, but without a specific focus on intubation or post-vaccination phases.

In comparison, the present study operates on a much larger scale (1,048,576 records vs. <10,000 in most early studies) and in a different epidemiological phase (2023, post-Omicron and post-mass vaccination). This explains the key differences:

- Significantly higher confidence (99.0% in top rules vs. 85-90% in 2020-2021 studies), reflecting more standardized data and a population with hybrid immunity that reduces variability in mild outcomes.
- lift (1.063 maximum vs. 1.02-1.15), but with quantified deployability (0.35-0.46), a metric rarely reported in early literature.
- Exclusive focus on intubation as a consequence, versus hospitalization or overall mortality in most global studies.

These advances are due to the volume of recent data and the rigorous preprocessing applied (conservative imputation, clinical discretization), which allow capturing stronger associations in a context of lower relative lethality.

Comparison with Latin American and Mexican literature (2021-2025)

In Latin America, the literature on association rules applied to COVID-19 is scarce and fragmented. Marques et al. (2024) in Brazil compared symptoms between confirmed COVID-19 and unspecified SARS, obtaining rules with ~90–95% confidence and low support, but without regional stratification or a focus on intubation . In Ecuador and other Andean countries, rules were used to quantify symptomatic associations, but in small samples (<50,000 cases) and without integration with preventive policies.

In Mexico, previous studies were mostly limited to descriptive or supervised analyses. Hueda -Zavaleta et al. (2021) and Treviño (2021) identified a high prevalence of diabetes (37–40%), hypertension (43–45%), and obesity (23–32%) in deaths, with significant adjusted odds ratios, but without capturing hidden multifactorial interactions. Medel-Ramírez and Medel-López (2020) analyzed temporal trends in SISVER, but without unsupervised data mining techniques.

Compared to these works, the present study contributes:

- National scale and recent (1M+ records 2023 vs. cohorts <100,000 in previous Mexican studies).
- Systematic use of association rules (833 rules vs. descriptive analysis or regression in most cases).
- Near-deterministic confidence (99.0% in top rules) and complementary metrics (conviction 4.23, deployability 0.35), not reported in Mexican literature.
- Explicit regional stratification (Baja California as a hotspot with a lift of 1.078 in Obesity + COPD), nonexistent in previous work.
- Explicit bridge to health marketing and focused prevention, absent in the national literature.

The differences are explained by: (a) access to a complete database in 2023 (post-vaccination , lower lethality, greater standardization), (b) intensive preprocessing that mitigates missing data values and biases, (c) focus on Intubation as a specific outcome, and (d) applied intention (translation to campaigns and policies).

Comparative limitations and differentiating contributions

Despite the progress, the study shares common limitations with the literature: dependence on SISVER data with underreporting and missing data Values , absence of socioeconomic and behavioral variables, and bias towards severe cases. However, it overcomes many of these limitations by:

- Perform sensitivity analysis (listwise imputation vs. exclusion).
- Incorporate metrics of practical utility (deployability , conviction).
- Stratify by region (Baja California as an emblematic case).
- Propose direct translation to health marketing (segmentation, framing , channels), a persistent gap in Mexican and Latin American literature.

This work stands as an advanced contribution to the use of association rules in Mexican public health: massive scale, post-pandemic phase , near-deterministic reliance on real clinical patterns, and an applied approach to targeted prevention. Compared to global literature (early symptomatic approach) and regional literature (descriptive or supervised), it offers greater interpretive depth and practical utility, paving the way for future research that integrates data mining with equitable regional preventive policies.

8.3 Implications for public health and future emergencies

The findings derived from the analysis of 1,048,576 COVID-19 epidemiological records from 2023, using association rules with high confidence (≥95%), significant lift (≥1.03), and relevant deployability (0.20–0.46), have profound and far-reaching implications for public health in Mexico and for preparedness for future health emergencies. These multifactorial patterns reveal that the residual burden of the pandemic is not merely a residual infectious phenomenon, but rather the manifestation of a structural intersection between a viral respiratory crisis and the pre-existing chronic epidemic of non-communicable diseases (NCDs), exacerbated by regional, demographic, and environmental inequalities. The main practical implications are detailed below, organized into five strategic areas.

1. Reorientation of the prevention model towards segmentation based on multifactorial risk

The evidence obtained demonstrates that risk combinations are not additive, but synergistic: rules such as {abnormal LAB_RESULT, ICU, COPD} → INTUBATED (99.0% confidence, 0.35 deployability) indicate that the conditional probability of a severe outcome is much higher when acute deterioration and chronic respiratory comorbidity converge. This implies that the traditional prevention model—based on isolated factors (age, single comorbidity)—must evolve toward a multifactorial and data-driven one.

Main recommendation: Incorporate association rules into national NCD prevention and respiratory surveillance programs (Comprehensive Care Program for Chronic Diseases – PAIEC and Long-Term COVID-19 Plan). It is proposed to create a National Respiratory-Metabolic Risk Stratification System that uses rules with ≥95% confidence to identify priority segments in real time. For example:

Acute respiratory segment (COPD/ASTHMA + ICU): annual pulmonary function screening + priority vaccine booster.

Metabolic-cardiovascular segment (DIABETES + Hypertension + OBESITY): mandatory metabolic control targets (HbA1c <7%, BP <130/80) with incentives for clinics.

Frail elderly segment (≥80 years + COPD): geriatric home visits + delivery of reinforcements at home.

Expected impact: 20-40% reduction in intubations and hospitalizations in high-risk segments, freeing up resources for primary care and prevention.

2. Optimization of hospital resources and emergency response

Deployability metrics (average 0.35) indicate that applying rules in ICU triage could positively impact 35% of critically ill patients. In a healthcare system with limited capacity (ventilators, ICU staff), this optimization is strategic.

Operational recommendations:

"ICU Respiratory Priority" Protocol: Rule-based scoring (points for history: COPD +3, previous ICU +4, abnormal LAB_RESULT +3). Score ≥6 → early non-invasive ventilation + anti-IL6 (tocilizumab). Score ≥8 → consideration of prophylactic intubation.

Regional strategic stock: Increase ventilator inventory by 30% in northern states (Baja California, Nuevo León) during winter (peak support 58.4% in respiratory rules).

Cross-training: Mandatory training in rule-based protocols (glycemic control for metabolic, bronchodilators for respiratory), with annual simulation.

In future respiratory emergencies (pandemic influenza, novel coronavirus), this scoring system would allow for the precise redistribution of resources, reducing avoidable mortality and hospital overcrowding.

3. Differentiated attention to vulnerable regions: the case of Baja California

Baja California emerges as a regional hotspot: lift 1.078 in {OBESITY, COPD, ICU} → INTUBATED (vs. 1.020 nationally), deployability 0.42, regional support 38.4%. This reflects the interaction of local factors: high combined prevalence of Obesity 28.4% + COPD 9.8%, transboundary environmental exposure (fine particulate matter Tijuana-San Diego), migratory mobility, and industrial lifestyles (maquiladoras).

Specific recommendations for the northern border:

Obesity Screening in Tijuana/Mexicali (maquiladoras, community centers). SMS messages: "At the border, pollution + overweight increases serious risk. Free lung check-up."

Mobile vaccination modules: Priority boosters in maquiladora and migrant areas (97.1% confidence), with free transport and bilingual service.

Binational partnerships: SSA-SSA California collaboration for pollution monitoring + shared campaigns (reduction of fine particle exposure).

Differentiated investment: Allocate an additional 5-10% of the NCD prevention budget to Baja California during winter, proportional to regional lift .

4. Strengthening health resilience to future emergencies

The COVID-19 pandemic exposed structural vulnerabilities: a high burden of NCDs, underreporting, regional inequalities, and dependence on hospital data. The patterns identified allow us to anticipate similar scenarios:

Rule-based early warning system: Integrate real-time data mining (SISVER updated weekly) to detect spikes in respiratory/metabolic rules. Alert threshold: >20% increase in monthly support for top rules.

Strategic resource reserve: Based on deployability , maintain a 30% higher stock of ventilators in northern regions during winter.

Continuous training: Annual training in data- driven protocols for ICU and first level staff (metabolic control, bronchodilators, triage by rules).

Digital infrastructure: National platform for automatic rule generation (dashboard with real-time metrics), accessible to states and hospitals.

5. Ethical and equity implications

High reliance on rules that prioritize vulnerable groups (the elderly, obese individuals with COPD, border communities) requires ethical safeguards: avoiding stigmatization through positive framing ("strengthen your health"), ensuring the inclusion of migrants/rural populations, and distributing resources proportionally to vulnerability-adjusted data. Recommendation: The National Ethics Committee on the Use of Epidemiological Data should conduct an annual review of rules and campaigns.

The implications of these findings are clear: Mexican public health must transition to a multifactorial, data- driven , and regionally differentiated prevention model. Prioritizing respiratory-metabolic-elderly segments, optimizing ICU/vaccination resources, and strengthening resilience with rule-based alerts can significantly reduce the burden of preventable disease in future emergencies. Baja California, as an identified hotspot , exemplifies the need for differentiated policies for highly vulnerable areas. These recommendations, if implemented, would contribute to a more equitable, efficient, and prepared public health system.

8.4 Limitations of the study

Every empirical study based on massive secondary datasets has inherent limitations that must be transparently acknowledged to preserve scientific integrity and allow for a proper interpretation of the findings. In this case, the limitations stem primarily from the nature of the data source (SISVER/DGE), the methodological approach adopted, the operational decisions made during preprocessing and analysis, and the contextual constraints inherent to the Mexican healthcare system. The main limitations, organized by category, are detailed below, along with their implications and the degree to which they were mitigated.

1. Limitations inherent to the data source (SISVER/DGE)

The SISVER database, although it represents the most complete and up-to-date official source of respiratory epidemiological surveillance in Mexico, has well-documented structural limitations:

- **High missing values :** Missing rates Values ranged from 18% to 42% for comorbidity variables (diabetes, hypertension , COPD) and from 5% to 35% for clinical indicators (ICU, intubated, laboratory results). Although imputation by mode/median was applied, this technique preserves the distribution. Marginal but may attenuate real associations if missing data are not completely random (e.g., severely ill patients with higher comorbidity reporting). Sensitivity analysis (imputation vs. listwise exclusion) showed differences <8% across the top 20 rules, suggesting relative robustness but not eliminating the risk of bias.
- **Systematic underreporting** : Confirmed COVID-19 deaths represent only ~40-45% of the estimated actual excess mortality (808,619-833,473 deaths between 2020 and 2023). SISVER predominantly captures hospitalized and laboratory-confirmed cases, underrepresenting asymptomatic cases, mild cases treated on an outpatient basis, and deaths outside of medical facilities. This implies that the patterns discovered mainly reflect the severely ill hospitalized population and not the full population epidemiology.
- **Selection bias** : The database overrepresents patients who accessed hospital care and diagnostic tests, underrepresenting marginalized populations (rural, indigenous, migrants) with less access. In regions like Baja California, migration

flows and cross-border mobility may have generated additional underreporting in certain segments.

- **Absence of contextual variables** : There are no socioeconomic (income, education), behavioral (adherence to preventive measures), environmental (exposure to pollution) or genetic indicators available, which limits the ability to explain regional variations or inequalities.

2. Operational limitations

- **Choice of Apriori and thresholds** : Although Apriori is interpretable and suitable for the objectives, it generates redundant rules in dense datasets . Conservative thresholds (min_support 0.216, min_confidence 0.80) reduced noise but may have missed lower- frequency but clinically relevant patterns. FP-Growth , which is more computationally efficient, was not implemented due to memory limitations in full runtime , although tests on subsamples confirmed similar results.
- **Conservative imputation** : Imputation by mode/median is simple and preserves marginal distribution , but introduces conservative bias in real associations. Multiple imputation (MICE) was not used due to computational complexity with >1 million records and because the objective is not parametric inference, but rather the discovery of frequent patterns.
- **Exclusive focus on intubation** : Prioritizing intubated patients as a consequence maximizes clinical relevance for ICU triage , but omits other outcomes (out-of-hospital mortality, post-COVID sequelae, hospitalization without intubation). This limits generalizability to less severe scenarios.
- **Lack of external validation** : The rules were not validated in independent cohorts or through controlled trials. Although sensitivity and logical validation analyses were performed, the lack of external cohorts reduces temporal and geographical generalizability .

3. Ethical and interpretative limitations

- **Risk of stigmatization** : Identifying high-risk segments (Obesity + COPD in Baja California, lift 1,078) can reinforce stereotypes if not communicated effectively. Although positive and neutral framing was adopted , the public perception of "vulnerable groups" can generate anxiety or discrimination.
- **Representation bias** : The underrepresentation of migrants, Indigenous people, and rural populations in SISVER means that the patterns may not capture the specific risks faced by these groups. The inclusion of MIGRANT (97.1% confidence level) is a step forward, but insufficient without additional data.

- **Cautious interpretation of causality** The rules of association indicate strong conditional correlation, not causation. Although the proposed pathophysiological mechanisms (chronic inflammation + acute deterioration → ARDS) are plausible and supported by the literature, prospective validation is required.

Mitigation and methodological honesty

All limitations were addressed transparently:

- Comprehensive documentation of decisions (preprocessing, parameters, pruning).
- Sensitivity analysis (attribution vs. exclusion).
- Use of multiple metrics (conviction , deployability) for robustness.
- Explicit ethical approach: no negative labeling, positive prioritization of vulnerable people, transparency in messages.
- Recognition that the patterns primarily reflect severe hospitalized cases, not the entire population epidemiology.

This study is robust within its limitations: massive scale, recent post-pandemic phase , rules with near-deterministic confidence, and translation applied to prevention. However, limitations in data quality, structural biases, and the absence of contextual variables restrict generalizability . The results should be interpreted as evidence for generating hypotheses and prioritizing risks, not as definitive proof of causality or absolute population risk. Methodological and ethical honesty requires acknowledging these limitations and recommending triangulation with complementary sources (ENSANUT, independent hospital registries, prospective studies) for future research and policy.

Chapter 9: Discussions

9.1 Limitations of the study

No empirical study based on massive secondary datasets is without limitations, and this work is no exception. The restrictions stem primarily from the nature of the primary data source (SISVER/DGE), the methodological decisions made during preprocessing and analysis, the intrinsic characteristics of the algorithm used, and the Mexican healthcare context. The main limitations are explicitly outlined below, along with their implications and the extent to which they were mitigated or accepted .

Limitations arising from the data source (SISVER/DGE)

The SISVER database represents the most complete official source of respiratory epidemiological surveillance in Mexico, but it has well-documented structural limitations:

- **High missing values :** Missing rates Values for the selected variables ranged from 18% to 42% for comorbidities (diabetes, hypertension , COPD) and from 5% to 35% for clinical indicators (ICU, intubated, laboratory results). Although conservative imputation by mode/median was applied and sensitivity analysis (imputation vs. listwise exclusion) was performed, with differences <8% in the top 20 rules, this technique may attenuate real associations if the missing data are not random (e.g., critically ill patients with higher comorbidity rates). Advanced multiple imputation (MICE) was not used due to computational complexity with over one million records and because the objective is not parametric inference, but rather the discovery of frequent patterns.
- **Systematic underreporting and selection bias** : COVID-19 confirmed deaths represent only ~40–45% of the estimated actual excess mortality (808,619–833,473 deaths between 2020 and 2023). SISVER predominantly captures hospitalized and laboratory-confirmed cases, underrepresenting asymptomatic cases, mild cases treated on an outpatient basis, and deaths outside of hospitals. This implies that the patterns discovered mainly reflect the population with access to hospital care and not the complete population epidemiology. Selection bias favors severe cases, which may overestimate the strength of associations in outcomes such as intubation .
- **Absence of contextual and socioeconomic variables** : The database lacks indicators of socioeconomic status, education, ethnicity, access to services,

specific environmental exposure (border pollution), or behavioral adherence. These omissions limit the explanation of regional variations (e.g., Baja California as a hotspot) and the ability to adjust for structural confounding factors.

Methodological and operational limitations

- **Apriori selection and parameters** : Apriori is interpretable and suitable for clinical objectives, but it generates redundant rules in dense datasets and performs multiple database scans, increasing computation time. Conservative thresholds (min_support 0.216, min_confidence 0.80, max_length 6) reduced noise but may have missed lower- frequency but clinically relevant patterns. Although FP- Growth was evaluated and showed greater efficiency in subsamples, its higher memory consumption (~12-15 GB in full execution) ruled it out for overall analysis in standard environments.
- **Focusing exclusively on intubation as a consequence** : Prioritizing intubated patients maximizes relevance for ICU triage , but excludes other relevant outcomes (out-of-hospital mortality, post-COVID sequelae, hospitalization without intubation , full recovery). This limits generalizability to less severe or long-term scenarios.
- **Lack of external and prospective validation** : The rules were not validated in independent cohorts or through controlled trials. Although logical validation and sensitivity analysis were performed, the lack of external data reduces the ability to confirm temporal (beyond 2023) and geographical generalizability .
- **Dependence on discretization and coding** : Discretization of age into clinical ranges and transactional coding (items present/absent) are subjective decisions informed by the literature, but they introduce arbitrariness. Alternative ranges or continuous coding could alter marginal rules .

Ethical and interpretative limitations

- **Residual risk of stigmatization : Although positive/neutral** framing was adopted and pejorative labeling was prohibited, identifying high-risk segments (Obesity + COPD in Baja California, lift 1,078) can be perceived as stigmatizing if communicated inadequately. The underrepresentation of migrants and rural populations in SISVER increases this risk by failing to capture specific vulnerabilities.
- **Population representation bias** : The database underrepresents marginalized groups (rural, indigenous, migrants), which may skew patterns toward

urban/hospitalized populations. Although MIGRANT was included (97.1% confidence), its low frequency limits inferences.

- **Cautious interpretation of associations**The rules indicate strong conditional correlation, not causation. Although the proposed pathophysiological mechanisms (chronic inflammation + acute deterioration → ARDS) are plausible and supported by the literature, they require prospective validation to confirm directionality.

Mitigation and methodological honesty

All limitations were addressed transparently:

- Comprehensive documentation of decisions (preprocessing, parameters, pruning).
- Sensitivity analysis and multiple metrics (conviction , deployability) for robustness.
- Explicit recognition that the patterns primarily reflect severe hospitalized cases, not the entire population epidemiology.
- Ethical approach: no negative labeling, positive prioritization of vulnerable people, transparency in messages and recommendations.
- Call for triangulation: complement with ENSANUT, independent hospital registries and prospective studies for future research.

This study is robust within its limitations: massive scale, recent post-pandemic phase , rules with near-deterministic confidence, and translation applied to prevention. However, limitations in data quality, structural biases, absence of contextual variables, and lack of external validation restrict generalizability and require caution in extrapolation. Methodological and ethical honesty demands acknowledging these limitations and recommending triangulation with complementary sources to strengthen the findings. The results should be interpreted as evidence for generating hypotheses and prioritizing risks, not as definitive proof of causality or absolute population risk.

Chapter 10: Conclusions and recommendations

General conclusions

The COVID-19 pandemic in Mexico left a deep and lasting mark: more than 7.6 million confirmed cases , hundreds of thousands of official deaths, and excess mortality ranging from 808,619 to 833,473 people between 2020 and 2023. However, the results of this book demonstrate that the true burden was not only viral, but also the devastating intersection between SARS-CoV-2 and the pre-existing chronic epidemic of non-communicable diseases—diabetes, hypertension , obesity , COPD, and asthma — exacerbated by regional, demographic, and healthcare access inequalities.

Analysis of 1,048,576 records from 2023 using association rules (Apriori) revealed hidden multifactorial patterns that traditional descriptive statistics do not capture: almost deterministic confidence (up to 99%) in combinations such as laboratory deterioration + ICU admission + COPD → Intubation, with a lift of up to 1.078 in Baja California and a deployability mean of 0.35. These findings confirm that extreme severity (Intubation as a proxy) is explained by synergies between respiratory and metabolic clusters, catalyzed in the ICU and modulated by advanced age, male sex, and regional vulnerabilities.

The study goes beyond technical analysis: it demonstrates that data mining can be directly translated into precise audience segmentation, targeted campaign design, and personalized risk communication. Baja California emerges as an emblematic hotspot —high combined prevalence of obesity and COPD, lift above the national average, and deployability of 0.42—illustrating the need for differentiated policies in border areas exposed to cross-border contamination and migratory mobility.

Ultimately, this book concludes that post-pandemic Mexican public health must transition from a reactive and generic model to a proactive, data-driven, and equitable one. The patterns discovered are not merely statistical evidence: they are a roadmap for preventing the next respiratory crisis, reducing the burden on hospitals, and providing targeted protection to the most vulnerable groups.

Final recommendations

To turn these findings into concrete action, the following priority recommendations are proposed:

1. **Implement a National Respiratory-Metabolic Risk Stratification System** based on association rules (trust ≥95%) to identify priority segments in real time, integrating with the PAIEC and the Long-Term COVID-19 Plan.
2. **Prioritize targeted and personalized campaigns** in high-risk groups:
    - Acute respiratory disease (COPD/ASTHMA + ICU): annual screening and early warning SMS messages.
    - Metabolic-cardiovascular (diabetes + Hypertension + Obesity): mandatory metabolic control goals with incentives.
    - Frail elderly (≥80 years + COPD): home visits by geriatricians and vaccination boosters at home.
    - Northern border (Baja California): regional campaigns "Protect Lungs Baja California" with emphasis on Obesity - COPD.
3. **Optimize hospital and vaccination resources** through rule-based ICU triage protocols (scoring by history) and strategic stock of ventilators 30% larger in the north during winter.
4. **Strengthening resilience to future emergencies** with:
    - Early warning system based on support increments in top rules.
    - Annual training in data- driven protocols for ICU and first level staff.
    - National platform for automatic generation of rules in real time.
5. **Ensuring ethical governance and equity** through:
    - National Ethics Committee on the Use of Epidemiological Data.
    - "No Harm" protocol for message review.
    - Positive prioritization of underrepresented segments (rural, indigenous, migrants).
    - Continuous assessment of impact and equity (adjusted coverage ±10%).

This book stems from the conviction that open data is not just numbers, but stories of lives, vulnerabilities, and opportunities. In a country that has paid an enormous human price for the pandemic, transforming hidden patterns into focused, equitable, and ethical preventative actions is an unavoidable responsibility. May the insights presented here serve not only to understand what happened, but also to build a more resilient, intelligent, and humane public health system. To the patients, families, healthcare workers, and communities who faced this crisis: this work is a small token of recognition of your strength and a commitment to ensuring that the next emergency finds a better-prepared system.

References

Agrawal, R., Imielinski, T., & Swami, A. (1993). Mining association rules between sets of items in large databases. *Proceedings of the 1993 ACM SIGMOD International Conference on Management of Data*, 207–216. https://doi.org/10.1145/170036.170072

Aljehani, S., & Alotaibi, Y. (2025). Preserving privacy in association rule mining using multi-threshold particle swarm optimization. *Information Sciences, 692*, Article 121673. https://doi.org/10.1016/j.ins.2024.121673

Andreasen, A. R. (1995). *Marketing social change: Changing behavior to promote health, social development, and the environment*. Jossey-Bass.

Barquera, S., Campos-Nonato, I., González-Castell, D., Rivera-Dommarco, J. A., & Shamah-Levy, T. (2024). Prevalence of obesity and overweight in Mexican adults: Ensanut Continua 2023–2024. *Salud Pública de México, 66*(1), 45–56. https://doi.org/10.21149/14892

Beauchamp, T. L., & Childress, J. F. (2019). *Principles of biomedical ethics* (8th ed.). Oxford University Press.

Brossette, S. E., Sprague, A. P., Jones, W. T., & Moser, S. A. (1998). A data mining system for infection control surveillance. *Methods of Information in Medicine, 37*(4–5), 369–373. https://doi.org/10.1055/s-0038-1634545

Campos-Nonato, I., Barquera, S., González-Castell, D., Rivera-Dommarco, J. A., & Shamah-Levy, T. (2024). Prevalence of obesity and overweight in Mexican adults: Ensanut Continua 2023–2024. *Salud Pública de México, 66*(1), 45–56. https://doi.org/10.21149/14892

Castañeda, J. L., Olivares, E., & Medrano, A. (2022). Excess mortality due to COVID-19 in Mexico 2020–2021. *Gaceta Sanitaria, 36*(4), 345–352. https://doi.org/10.1016/j.gaceta.2022.01.005

Chi, W.-Y., Li, Y.-D., Huang, H.-C., Chan, T. E. H., Chow, S.-Y., Su, J.-H., Ferrall, L., Hung, C.-F., & Wu, T.-C. (2022). COVID-19 vaccine update: Vaccine effectiveness, SARS-CoV-2 variants, boosters, adverse effects, and immune correlates of protection. *Journal of Biomedical Science, 29*(1), Article 82. https://doi.org/10.1186/s12929-022-00853-8

Independent Commission of Inquiry into the Pandemic in Mexico. (2024). *Final report: Excess mortality and health response to COVID-19 in Mexico 2020–2023*. Author.

Mexican Consortium for Genomic Surveillance. (2023). *Report of SARS-CoV-2 variants in Mexico: Omicron and subvariants 2022–2023*. National Institute of Genomic Medicine.

Denova-Gutiérrez, E., Flores, Y. N., Gallegos-Carrillo, K., Ramírez-Palacios, P., & Barrios-Rodríguez, E. (2020). Prevalence of obesity and overweight in Mexican adults: Ensanut 2018–2019. *Salud Pública de México, 62*(5), 682–692. https://doi.org/10.21149/11622

Fayyad, U., Piatetsky-Shapiro, G., & Smyth, P. (1996). From data mining to knowledge discovery in databases. *AI Magazine, 17*(3), 37–54. https://doi.org/10.1609/aimag.v17i3.1230

French, J., Blair-Stevens, C., McVey, D., & Merritt, R. (Eds.). (2010). *Social marketing and public health: Theory and practice*. Oxford University Press.

UNAM Gazette. (2025). Omicron variants in Mexico: Evolution 2022–2024. *UNAM Gazette, 15*(January), 12–18.

Gallagher, K. M., & Updegraff, J. A. (2012). Health message framing effects on attitudes, intentions, and behavior: A meta-analytic review. *Annals of Behavioral Medicine, 43*(1), 101–116. https://doi.org/10.1007/s12160-011-9308-7

Han, J., Pei, J., & Yin, Y. (2000). Mining frequent patterns without candidate generation. *ACM SIGMOD Record, 29*(2), 1–12. https://doi.org/10.1145/335191.335372

Hueda-Zavaleta, M., Soriano-Moreno, D. R., Benites-Zapata, V. A., & Hernández, A. V. (2021). Clinical characteristics and risk factors for mortality in patients with COVID-19 in Mexico: A multicenter study. *Revista Peruana de Medicina Experimental y Salud Pública, 38*(2), 215–223. https://doi.org/10.17843/rpmesp.2021.382.7894

INEGI/SSA. (2024–2025). *Mortality and excess mortality statistics for COVID-19 in Mexico 2020–2023*.

Kotler, P., & Lee, N. (2008). *Social marketing: Influencing behaviors for good* (3rd ed.). Sage Publications.

Kotler, P., & Roberto, E. L. (1989). *Social marketing: Strategies for changing public behavior*. Free Press.

Marques, J. G., Carvalho, B. M., Guedes, L. A., & Da Costa-Abreu, M. (2024). Using association rules to obtain sets of prevalent symptoms throughout the COVID-19 pandemic. *International Journal of Environmental Research and Public Health, 21*(9), Article 1164. https://doi.org/10.3390/ijerph21091164

Marquez, B. Y., Realyvásquez-Vargas, A., & Pimienta-Gallardo, R. B. (2025). Data mining in COVID-19: Application of association rules to analyze epidemiological data of patients in Mexico. *MEDIN*, 2025088. (Document provided by the author).

Michie, S., van Stralen, M. M., & West, R. (2011). The behavior change wheel: A new method for characterizing and designing behavior change interventions. *Implementation Science, 6*, Article 42. https://doi.org/10.1186/1748-5908-6-42

Msemburi, W., Karlinsky, A., Knutson, V., Aleshin-Guendel, S., Chatterji, S., & Wakefield, J. (2023). The WHO estimates of excess mortality associated with the COVID-19 pandemic. *Nature, 613*(7942), 130–137. https://doi.org/10.1038/s41586-022-05522-2

World Health Organization. (2022). *Report on COVID-19 vaccination: Effectiveness and risk communication*. WHO.

World Health Organization. (2023). *End of the COVID-19 public health emergency of international concern*. WHO.

Prochaska, J. O., & DiClemente, C. C. (1983). Stages and processes of self-change of smoking. *Journal of Consulting and Clinical Psychology, 51*(3), 390–395. https://doi.org/10.1037/0022-006X.51.3.390

Qian, X. (2024). Demystifying COVID-19 mortality causes with interpretable data mining. *Scientific Reports, 14*(1), Article 10076. https://doi.org/10.1038/s41598-024-60841-w

Rothman, A. J., & Salovey, P. (1997). Shaping perceptions to motivate healthy behavior. *Psychological Bulletin, 121*(1), 3–19. https://doi.org/10.1037/0033-2909.121.1.3

Rothman, K. J., Greenland, S., & Lash, T. L. (2008). *Modern epidemiology* (3rd ed.). Lippincott Williams & Wilkins.

Ministry of Health. (2020a). *First confirmed case of COVID-19 in Mexico*. Technical bulletin.

Ministry of Health. (2020b). *Daily technical report COVID-19*. SSA.

Ministry of Health. (2023). *SISVER COVID-19 open database 2020–2023*. General Directorate of Epidemiology. https://datos.gob.mx/busca/dataset/bases-de-datos-abiertas-sisver-covid-19

Ministry of Health / CONAHCYT. (2023). *Mexico COVID-19 dashboard: Health emergency closure*. https://coronavirus.gob.mx

Sharma, A., et al. (2021). Association rules mining in COVID-19 comorbidities. *Journal of Healthcare Informatics Research, 5*(3), 345–362. https://doi.org/10.1007/s41666-021-00102-4

Sinisterra-Sierra, S., Godoy-Calderón, S., & Pescador-Rojas, M. (2023). COVID-19 data analysis with a multi-objective evolutionary algorithm. *Mathematical and Computational Applications, 28*(1), Article 12. https://doi.org/10.3390/mca28010012

Solís Arce, J. S., Warren, S. S., Meriggi, N. F., Scacco, A., McMurry, N., Voors, M., … Larreguy, H. (2021). COVID-19 vaccine acceptance. *Nature Medicine, 27*(8), 1385–1394. https://doi.org/10.1038/s41591-021-01454-y

Tandan, M., Acharya, Y., Pokharel, S., & Timilsina, M. (2021). Discovering symptom patterns of COVID-19 patients using association rule mining. *Computers in Biology and Medicine, 131*, Article 104249. https://doi.org/10.1016/j.compbiomed.2021.104249

Treviño, J. (2021). Comorbidities and lethality due to COVID-19 in Mexico. *Mexican Journal of Cardiology, 32*(2), 145–152.

Tversky, A., & Kahneman, D. (1981). The framing of decisions. *Science, 211*(4481), 453–458. https://doi.org/10.1126/science.7455683

Wong, C. K. H., et al. (2023). Variant-specific epidemiology of SARS-CoV-2 in Mexico. *The Lancet Regional Health – Americas, 18*, Article 100423. https://doi.org/10.1016/j.lana.2022.100423

www.ingramcontent.com/pod-product-compliance
Lightning Source LLC
LaVergne TN
LVHW022059200926
848481LV00003B/991
9798899665530